The Musician's Hand

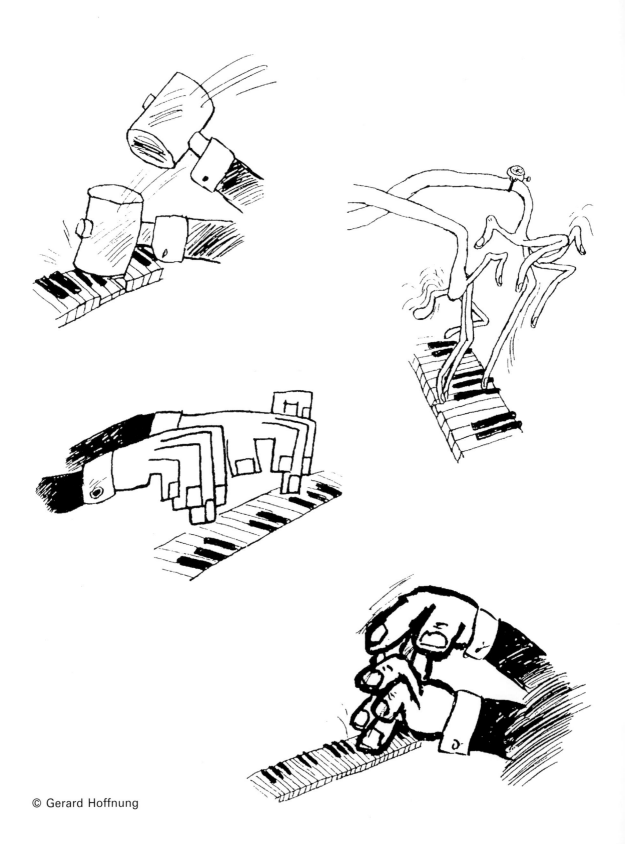

The Musician's Hand
A Clinical Guide

Edited by

Ian Winspur FRCS, FACS

Christopher B Wynn Parry MBE, MA, DM, FRCP, FRCS

The Hand Clinic
Devonshire Hospital
London, UK

MARTIN ■ DUNITZ

First published in the United Kingdom in 1998 by
Martin Dunitz Ltd
The Livery House
7–9 Pratt Street
London NW1 0AE

A CIP record for this book is available from the British Library.

ISBN 1 85317 492 0

Distributed in the United States by:
Blackwell Science Inc.
Commerce Place, 350 Main Street
Malden, MA 02148, USA
Tel: 1-800-215-1000

Distributed in Canada by:
Login Brothers Book Company
324 Salteaux Crescent
Winnipeg, Manitoba, R3J 3T2
Canada
Tel: 204-224-4068

Distributed in Brazil by:
Ernesto Reichmann Distribuidora de Livros, Ltda
Rua Coronel Marques 335, Tatuape 03440-000
Sao Paulo,
Brazil

Composition by Scribe Design, Gillingham, Kent, UK
Printed and bound in Spain by Grafos

CONTENTS

LIST OF CONTRIBUTORS

Yves Allieu
Service de Chirurgie Orthopédique et Trauma-
tologique II
Hôpital Lapeyronie
F-34295 Montpellier Cedex 5, France

Peter C Amadio
Orthopedic Surgery
Mayo Clinic
200 First Street SW
Rochester, Minnesota 55905, USA

Yolande Baeten
Service de Chirurgie Orthopédique et
Traumatologique II
Hôpital Lapeyronie
F-34295 Montpellier Cedex 5, France

Alison T Davis
Hand Therapy Unit
King Edward VII Hospital
Midhurst
West Sussex GU29 0BL, UK

Andy Evans
Arts Psychology Consultants
29 Argyll Mansions
Hammersmith Road
London W14 8QQ, UK

Simon Fischer
Guildhall School of Music and Drama
Barbican Centre
Silk Street
London EC2, UK

Bernard Gregor-Smith
Cellist of the Lindsay String Quartet
Manchester University
Manchester, UK

Carola Grindea
Performing Arts Clinic
28 Emperor's Gate
London SW7 4HS, UK

Kamel Hamitouche
Service de Chirurgie Orthopédique et
Traumatologique II
Hôpital Lapeyronie
F-34295 Montpellier Cedex 5, France

Geoffrey Hooper
Princess Margaret Rose Orthopaedic
Hospital
41–43 Frogston Road West
Edinburgh EH10 7ED, UK

Ian James
Department of Medicine
Royal Free Hospital
Pond Street
London NW3 2QG, UK

Jane Kember
The Elgin Physiotherapy Clinic
4 Elgin Road
Alexandra Park
London N22 4EU, UK

Geoffrey Leader
Department of Anaesthesia
Devonshire Hospital
29–31 Devonshire Road
London W1N 1RF, UK

Robert E Markison
Medical Arts Building
2000 Van Ness Avenue, Suite 502
San Francisco, California 94109–3017, USA

Jean Pillet
32, rue Godot de Mauroy
F-75009 Paris, France

Gabriele Rogers
Hand Therapy Unit
Devonshire Hospital
29–31 Devonshire Street
London W1N 1RF, UK

Jean-Luc Roux
Service de Chirurgie Orthopédique et
Traumatologique II
Hôpital Lapeyronie
F-34295 Montpellier Cedex 5, France

Helen Scott
Department of Occupational Therapy
Princess Margaret Rose Orthopaedic Hospital
41–43 Frogston Road West
Edinburgh EH10 7ED, UK

John Stanley
Centre for Hand and Upper Limb Surgery
Wrightington Hospital for Joint Disease
Hall Lane, Appley Bridge
Wigan WN6 9EP, UK

Hellmut Stern
Ass. Concertmaster and Chairman of
The Board of Musicians (retd)
Berlin Philharmonic Orchestra
Matthäikirchstr. 1
10785 Berlin, Germany

Raoul Tubiana
Institut de la Main
6, square Jouvenet
F-75016 Paris, France

Stewart Watson
Plastic Surgery Unit
Withington Hospital
Nell Lane, Didsbury
Manchester M20 8LR, UK

John Williams
c/o Harold Holt
31 Sinclair Rd
London W14 0NS

Ian Winspur
Hand Clinic
Devonshire Hospital
29–31 Devonshire Street
London W1N 1RF, UK

Christopher B Wynn Parry
Department of Rehabilitation
Devonshire Hospital
29–31 Devonshire Street
London W1N 1RF, UK

ACKNOWLEDGEMENTS

A number of the illustrations have been kindly provided by sources other than the contributing author for the text:

Frontispiece drawings by Gerard Hoffnung. Reproduced by courtesy of Annetta Hoffnung;

Figs 2 and 3a,b in Chapter 3 are by courtesy of All Flutes Plus, London;

Fig. 6 in Chapter 6 and Figs 3, 6 and 7 in Chapter 10 are by courtesy of Dr G Crawford;

Fig. 16 in Chapter 7 is by courtesy of Michael Freyham;

Figs 4a,b in Chapter 3 are by courtesy of JP Guiver & Co., London;

Fig. 9b in Chapter 10 is by courtesy of K Harrison;

Fig. 3 in Chapter 2 is by courtesy of Howarth of London;

Fig. 20 in Chapter 7 is by courtesy of L Murray, RGN;

Figs 6-11 in Chapter 3 are by courtesy of M de Gori

Fig. 8 in Chapter 9 is redrawn from A Narakas (p. 365) in R Tubiana, ed. *The Hand*, vol. 4. WB Saunders: Philadelphia, 1993, with permission;

Figs 22, 23 and 24 in Chapter 7 are by courtesy of Dr D Phelps;

Fig. 1 in Chapter 2, Fig. 1 in Chapter 3, Figs 1 and 3 in Chapter 5 and Fig 9 in Chapter 9 are by courtesy of Dr ABM Rietveld;

Figs 1a,b,c in Chapter 7 and Fig. 4 in Chapter 8 are by courtesy of Dr J Riley;

Figs 4 in Chapter 6, 18 in Chapter 7, and 6 in Chapter 9 are from pp. 276, 296 and 171 in R Tubiana, CJ McCullough, AC Masquelet, *An Atlas of Surgical Exposures of the Upper Extremity*. Martin Dunitz and JB Lippincott: London and Philadelphia, 1990;

Fig. 2 in Chapter 10 is redrawn from I Winspur (p. 23) in JA Bostwick, ed. *Current Concepts in Hand Surgery*. Lea & Febiger: Philadelphia, 1983, with permission;

Fig. 2 in Chapter 5 is from Winspur I, Wynn Parry CB (1997). The Musician's Hand. *J. Hand Surg* **22B**:433–40;

Fig. 1 in Chapter 13 is from P Brand. Mechanics of individual muscles at individual joints. In: *Clinical Mechanics of the Hand*. Mosby: St Louis, 1985, pp. 192–309.

FOREWORD

Why has there been a sudden interest in musicians' medical problems when these problems are probably as old as music and medicine themselves?

For a long time, functional disorders in musicians were dismissed by doctors with no treatment available and, for convenience, were considered to be induced by psychological and emotional upset. Equally, musicians themselves have, for a long time, been reticent about admitting to being susceptible to disabilities to the detriment of their career. Only recently, have organic and neurological aetiologies been recognized, although the borders between the various conditions encountered are often still not clear.

This recent interest in medical problems in musicians is due to a combination of various factors:

1) The wide diversity of musical activities in most countries, encouraged by television and the media, which has considerably increased the number of these disorders.
2) The increase in the number of epidemiological studies showing the high incidence of medical problems in instrumentalist musicians.
3) The development of sports and occupational medicine and the identification of "overuse injuries" which has obvious similarities with the injuries of musicians.
4) The creation and development of a new medical discipline – performing arts medicine – and of medical centres specializing in the treatment of medical problems in musicians.

As most of these problems are caused by functional motor disorders, it seems necessary that performing artists and especially music teachers should have a basic knowledge of anatomy and physiology, subjects poorly covered in conservatories. They should learn the normal mechanism of movements in order to become aware of non-physiological movements. Athletes are in many ways comparable to musicians, as both are motivated to perform to the limits of their abilities, involving rapid, complex, co-ordinated movements; however, athletes have learned to develop their musculature symmetrically in association with the practice of more specific physical movements. This is not so for most musicians. Whilst athletes are constantly surrounded by trainers, soothed by masseurs and physiotherapists and supervised by specialists in sports medicine, musicians, who depend on perfect fitness, are left to their own devices.

Even though the hand or the mouth is the major tool of the musician, the whole body is affected by the posture adopted when playing. Musicians should remember that the spine and thoracic cage are the stabilizing bony units for upper limb movement. All segments of the skeleton are interdependent: movements away from the resting position provoke reactions elsewhere. Thus an exaggeration of the thoracic kyphosis causes a forward projection of the head and an excessive compensatory lordosis of the cervical spine, all of which are accompanied by various muscular and ligamentous tensions. The importance of "good posture" cannot be overstressed during music practice. But what is meant by "good posture"? It is a condition where the whole body is in physiological equilibrium and can avoid the use of muscle groups other than those required for a given movement. Good posture allows the repetitive specific movements with a minimum of stress to the body. Of course, whilst playing, it is impossible to avoid momentary lapses from an ideal posture, but one must not allow long-term imbalances to become established, as chronic poor posture is difficult to correct and is the main factor in severe disabilities. Of the editors in this book, Kit Wynn Parry has been a pioneer in rehabilitation whose book *Rehabilitation of the Hand* is a classic; together with Ian Winspur, he has, over the years, acquired an exceptional knowledge and experience in the treatment of problems in performing artists. This book not only deals with medical aspects but also reflects the passionate interest of the authors in the complex personalities of the artists. It will certainly be very useful not only for physicians and physiotherapists but also for music teachers and artists themselves.

Raoul Tubiana

PREFACE

An apology for this book from a physician and a surgeon is that we not only love music but believe it to be fundamental to civilized living.

Plato wrote that 'Education in music is most sovereign because more than anything else rhythm and harmony find their way to the soul inmost and take strongest hold upon it, imparting grace if one is rightly trained. Music reduces to order and harmony any disharmony in the revolutions within us.' The Greeks considered that instruction in singing and playing the lyre should be a regular part of education for every freeborn citizen. The tradition has been persistent: Handel remarked to Lord Kinoull after the first London performance of *Messiah* 'I should be sorry, my Lord, if I have succeeded in entertaining them – I wished to make them better.'

In a study of New York children aged 2–6 years who had played in Alexander Blackman's Orchestra, it was found that all the children who had had this opportunity were well ahead of their classmates in all subjects when they entered school. Dance, and therefore music, is fundamental in all traditional cultures. One has only to read *The songlines*, where Bruce Chatwin (1987) describes the way in which territorial boundaries and links with neighbouring tribes are sung and danced to realize the supreme importance of music as an integral part of social life.

In many countries, not least the United Kingdom, politicians have sidelined the Arts as tangential and far from fundamental to living. The steady withdrawal of funding for music in British schools is to be deplored, and the generation of musicians who benefited from the enlightened attitude to music in schools thirty years ago will not be duplicated if present attitudes to the Arts persist.

We wholeheartedly agree with Antony Storr (1992) when he says 'Music is a powerful instrument of education which can be used for good or ill and we should ensure that everyone in our society is given the opportunity in participating in a wide range of different kinds of music.' The philistinism of so much of Britain today could be transformed in one or two generations if every child were given the opportunity to play an instrument as part of school activities.

The kernel of this book is the medical and surgical care of the musician's hand. However, the whole of the upper extremity is necessarily discussed. Similarly, one cannot divorce the musician's physical problems from his or her lifestyle, temperament and psyche. Hence the many different aspects covered by the contents of this book.

We would like to thank the secretarial and editorial staff at Martin Dunitz and specifically Robert Peden and Clive Lawson for their gentle but firm guidance and help. We would like to thank all the contributors for their hard work inside deadlines. Finally, we would like to thank all musicians – friends, patients and performers – for providing the inspiration and encouragement to complete this book.

IW
CWP
London, 1997

Chatwin B (1987) *The songlines*, Jonathan Cape: London.

Storr A (1992) *Music and the mind*, Free Press: Riverside, NJ.

1
The musician's perspective

The orchestra

Hellmut Stern

Music the sublime art! How many happy hours it gives to the lucky listener. How it lets them escape from the mundane routine of everyday life. How it lifts their minds to higher regions. And how happy and lucky are those who are fortunate enough to play professionally. While others are rushing early in the morning to their work, musicians are able to play, seldom starting before 10.00 a.m. Their whole lives are spent playing and they even get paid for it! What a splendid, enviable existence. But there is the business of music. If one focuses more accurately, the happy picture of the musician seen by the uninitiated looks very different. I would like to illustrate a small segment of the musician's daily life. Because I am a violinist I will use, as an example, the career or an orchestral violinist.

It is very often the ambitious parents and later the music teachers who aspire to a brilliant musical career for the child. As a rule, little thought is given to the consequences the persistent one-sided burden has on the child from whom even at a tender age great achievements are expected. The physical and psychological effect this has on the aspiring professional musician is scarcely considered at this time.

From the beginning the child is exposed to pressure to perform. To learn the profession at all the child must start to study at an early age. At this stage the foundations for some later physical and mental disturbances and disadvantages are already being laid down. To start with the child and, in most cases, the parents are carelessly oblivious of this.

A violin career must begin at an early age. The child who would often rather play football with his contemporaries than the violin on his own finds himself under continually increasing pressure. The child must practise a great deal and there are many activities, sport for example, which they may not participate in for fear of injury to the hands. Inevitably, the child's social interrelationships are disturbed. Competitive thinking and behaviour develop early. The hopes of parents and teachers for a successful violin career induce potent psychological pressure. In addition, there is the scholastic curriculum and all its demands which intensify the workload.

The study of an extensive repertoire is an essential requirement and technical perfection a prerequisite for progress and success (school and conservatory exams, competitions, solo concerts, etc.). Due to the long and often arduous time invested, the career of the growing child is largely predetermined and other subjects are not taken into consideration. Indeed a change of orientation is often no longer possible. Because of many factors, different for each individual, most violinists do not reach the prized soloist career, but now they are no longer children and they are compelled to face reality. For many now follows the 'descent' into the orchestra.

To an outsider the orchestra may appear integrated and harmonious. In reality, however, it is a strict hierarchical structure, full of discordance. All string players are by function fundamentally 'Tuttisten' (that is to say they play almost always en bloc) and, except for the principal violinist, are only rarely individually heard. All other musical instruments, the woodwind, brass, timpani, percussion and harp, are independently heard. They are the 'soloists' of the orchestra. This distinction is as noticeable in the attitude of the conductor as it is in salary. The difference in status creates a mental inequality between orchestral members which affects their professional behaviour.

Being part of the orchestra requires constant suppression of unpleasant circumstances. Some of these circumstances may be avoidable and some unavoidable. Many are unreasonable. The way this is felt by each musician is different and each copes in different ways. A physical and psychological analysis of all aspects of the life and work of the orchestral musician is therefore of decisive importance if positive changes, solutions or even simple relief from stress are to be brought about.

I use one example from among the many inadequacies of the orchestral fabric which complicates the job of the string player and often leads to mental and physical complaints – the seating order in the orchestra. The strings need ample room for their arm movement. In contrast to their colleagues playing the woodwind, brass and percussion, who have their own music sheets and desk, two string players have to share one desk. On many stages, but especially in the orchestra pit, there is a great shortage of space, so that the freedom of movement of the string players is severely restricted. The fear of impeding one's colleague sitting on the right or left or even of touching him with the bow is irritating and hinders freedom of movement, thereby disturbing concentration.

The music must be read from the side, which often leads to differences between desk partners, especially if their vision differs. In contrast, all other colleagues have their music sheets directly in front of their eyes and, if they so please, they are able to seat themselves comfortably. Bad visibility plays a big role and leads to physical and mental complaints. If, for example, the podium or the orchestral pit light is weak, the fear of making mistakes increases because the music sheet and the notations indicating the bowing movements are difficult to see. One gets 'hung-up' on individual note or groups of notes and at those moments loses flexibility and the necessary quick reflexes.

The reflection of the light off pencil-written bow stroke notations and the unwelcome fingering notations of one's desk partner can also lead to great irritation. I must also mention here that the printing of music sheets is often of poor quality, which also imposes a burden on the violinist since he has to read the greatest number of notes. Another difficulty arises through varying heights. If the rear seats of the string section are not raised, the musician of small stature who is sitting behind a taller colleague obviously has difficulty seeing the conductor. In such a case, fear develops because visual contact with the conductor cannot be guaranteed. If seating is restricted, it is not always possible simply by moving one's chair to obtain a clear field of vision. One gets too close to one's neighbour and the music sheet once again has to be moved, which in turn can lead to disagreement with one's desk partner (I speak from bitter experience).

It can also happen that partners on the last desk of the first violins must sit behind the second violins. Since the two groups often have different bowing strokes, this also becomes very irritating and disturbs concentration.

In the confined orchestra pit, the rear desks of the string section are situated close beside and in front of the woodwind and sometimes even very near the brass and percussion. In works of Wagner, Strauss or Berg, to name but a few, the acoustic burden is so immense that one can no longer hear one's own instrument. Earache and headaches occur to the point of nausea. In situations like these ear protectors are used by many orchestral musicians. In as much as a high performance level is expected, this is unreasonable. After all, playing the violin requires more sensitivity than the service of a sledgehammer.

When several of the factors described coincide, a panic situation can ensue which can lead to serious and lasting disturbances of hearing, with hearing loss and tinnitus. These injuries are common among orchestral musicians. This can mean the end of professional life.

The examples given are well known to every string player in the orchestra. Usually light is made of these problems and they are dismissed as unavoidable side issues. Few, however, are conscious of the psychosomatic burden and damage this can cause in the course of a long orchestral career. A number of stress situations would disappear if the musicians, the conductors and the management would be prepared to show goodwill and jointly tackle structural reforms to remedy avoidable deficiencies.

Von Karajan demanded during the first filming of the complete Beethoven symphonies that the music stands be lowered to a uniform height of approximately 10 cm and the violinists' heads be held high. Naturally one had to squint downwards, which was very uncomfortable. In addition, all the bow tips had to move up and down in unison. All orchestra members with little or no hair had to wear wigs, which caused them to sweat heavily since the film lights, each 1000 watts, pointed directly at the violin group. This absurd, but true, example not only illustrates the problems, but also shows how life in the orchestra with its many facets, including and especially the omnipotence of the conductor, could become complicated to the point of the grotesque.

Editors' comment

In all fairness, one should note that orchestras have been known to demoralize a conductor for whom they have little liking or respect; more than one talented conductor has been broken thus by an unsympathetic orchestra.

Pop and rock musicians

Ian Winspur

Hellmut Stern has given us a witty but poignant insight into the psychological and physical problems which beset orchestral players. We know, however, that pop and rock musicians suffer similar, if not identical, types of physical and psychological problems, although the origins are different.

As children, aspiring pop and rock musicians do not suffer the same pressures as those children studying an instrument classically. However, as teenagers, particularly if successful, they are subject to enormous, confusing psychological pressure. Sandie Shaw, the British pop singer, from her own experience as a teenage pop idol and latterly from her experience as a psychologist working with young musicians recently gave a very moving lecture at a conference on musicians in medicine in York (Shaw 1998). She highlighted the difficulties which idolized teenage stars have in maturing into adults both psychologically and

musically. Surrounded by adoring fans, sycophantic agents and record executives and manipulative managers, their life is an unreal one. Their world has no normal values. Their every antic is treated with approbation. They are encouraged to remain immature. And it is not surprising that when the cold light of the adult world strikes, perhaps when fashions have changed and success is waning, they are poorly equipped to cope. Physical disability may follow psychological decline.

Shaw also pointed out the difficulties the young pop star faces in trying to mature as a musician. If their records are selling, even if the artist sees that their current musical performance does not match their own developing skills and maturity, the music industry with its focus on established formulas and commercial success will try to limit any experimentation and change. She highlights George Michael as an example of one who, with an unusually mature and secure ego, through his own dogged determination helped by the financial security of earlier success, took on the record industry and won and was able, free of contracts, to evolve musically along his own lines. The majority of young pop and rock artists are unable to make this change and end up musically unfulfilled and dissatisfied and forced to endure the hardship of endless touring with a plethora of increasing psychological and physical problems.

Indeed the touring rock and pop musician may have an even harder physical existence than the orchestral player. The noise is immense and many have high-tone deafness and tinnitus. The gigs are late and the facilities poor, and the musicians themselves spend many hours carrying and lifting heavy amplification equipment and musical instruments. The gigs are often geographically far apart and therefore much time is spent sleeping in cars or buses or on aeroplanes with snatched late meals. Alcohol and drugs, producing artificial energy boosts and euphoria, provide temporary false relief. Poorly tuned instruments, particularly guitars tuned with excessive string tension, and equipment problems produce added strains.

Finally, many pop and rock guitarists are self-taught and their instrumental technique is flawed. When their playing is limited, this causes no difficulty, but with increasing success the playing demands increase. This is particularly so with long tours and in such circumstances upper body symptoms start to surface – aching arms, shoulder and neck pain and pain related to specific joints and digits. Poor playing patterns develop and indeed focal dystonias may also arise. They cannot seek help from their colleagues or managers for there are hungry replacements waiting on the side lines for their places in the band. The unfortunate young star soldiers on past a point where damage is being inflicted. With little psychological or emotional reserve and a lack of external support or help the decline can be rapid.

Reference

Shaw S (1998) Proceedings of the International Congress on Musicians: Health and the Musician. York 1997. British Association of Performing Arts Medicine: London.

2
The musician's hand and arm pain

Christopher B Wynn Parry

There is a crisis in the arts worldwide, although it is more acute in the United Kingdom, where sponsorship is declining, the government support of the arts is diminishing and in many orchestras the musician has no planned career structure or pension. Most musicians have to supplement their earnings with session work and teaching and many spend their life travelling from recording sessions, to rehearsals, to concerts to conservatories, arriving back home late at night with rushed, inadequate meals and no time to indulge in a healthy lifestyle with recreation and proper holidays. Added to which, there has been little or no training in schools or in music colleges as to care of the body and maintenance of a sensible lifestyle. Teachers on the whole are ignorant about ergonomics and the way the body works and do not give advice on the correct approach to a lifetime in music. Moreover, most academies and conservatoires are training musicians to be soloists, when the overwhelming majority, if they are lucky, will have a life in the rank and file of an orchestra.

Orchestral managers tell us that students arrive at the orchestra to start their career inadequately prepared, knowing very little of the repertory and with bad practice and performing habits. Tension within the orchestra and personal difficulties are well known, so that the life of the orchestral musician is full of physical, mental and emotional problems. It is surprising that more do not break down with stress-related illnesses and severe musculo-skeletal symptoms. Indeed, the various surveys show that the majority of musicians do have such problems, but because the musical career is so fraught, they are prepared to play with pain and suffer in silence. No musician wishes to share his problem with anyone else. There is a well recognized secrecy among the profession; it is important to the musician that orchestral managers and agents do not know of any such problems.

String and keyboard players have to make a remarkable number of repetitive movements in a short time with great accuracy. Paget studied Mademoiselle Genotha playing a presto by Mendelssohn on the piano. In 4 minutes, 3 seconds 5595 notes were played; 72 bimanual finger movements per second were recorded (Critchley and Henson 1977). It takes many years of practice to achieve dexterity and precision of this nature. The majority of musicians have to practise for many hours. On the face of it, there-fore, it is not surprising that many musicians complain of aches and pains in the upper limbs, particularly the hands and shoulders.

An explosion of interest in musicians' problems occurred in 1986 with the publication of the International Convention of Symphony and Orchestra Musicians' Survey in America (Fishbein et al 1988). A total of 4000 questionnaires were sent out – 56% of questionnaires were returned and some worrying statistics resulted. Overall 66% of string players recorded musculoskeletal problems, 48% of woodwind players and 32% of brass players. The shoulder, neck and lower back were particularly problematic locations among string players. In this group 16% reported a severe problem with the right shoulder and 14% with the left shoulder; 14% listed a problem with each side of the neck; 14% indicated a severe problem with the right lower back and 12% the left lower back. The left hand and the fingers of the left hand were naturally reported as having frequent symptoms. Twelve per cent of string players overall reported musculoskeletal problems severe enough to affect their performance. It was found that there were no gender differences among violinists, but there were significant gender differences among cellists, where females had many more problems than males.

Many other health problems were reported: 10% were worried about their smoking, 21% about their alcohol intake and 20% about the use of prescription and non-prescription drugs. Twenty-seven per cent of the musicians reported using betablockers at some stage and this was particularly prevalent among brass players. Finally, 24% of the musicians reported experiencing stage fright and stage fright was by far the most frequently mentioned problem after musculoskeletal problems. Psychological problems such as acute anxiety were reported by 13%, depression by 17% and sleep disturbances by 14%. Thus, overall 76% of musicians performing with these orchestras reported at least one medical problem that was severe in terms of its effect on performance.

At about this time Gary Graffman (Graffman 1986), a distinguished American pianist, reported his experience with dystonia in the journal *Medical Problems of Performing Artists*. He described graphically the lack of understanding and marked ignorance among the many medical specialists whom he consulted. As a result of this article, he was inundated with calls from fellow musicians all around America who had severe problems and were unable to get satisfaction from the medical profession. Musicians additionally have an almost pathological fear of doctors, let alone surgical intervention, and they were therefore routinely consulting practitioners of alternative medicine, so that it might be months or years before they came into the hands of orthodox physicians.

As a result of this publicity, clinics were set up in various parts of the world, particularly in the USA, the UK, France and Australia, and reports appeared on the incidence and nature of the problems presented. The clinical conditions frequently related to the specialty of the referring consultant, particularly in the USA. For example, neurologists reported a high incidence of dystonia and orthopaedic surgeons a high incidence of entrapment neuropathies, and rheumatologists frequently reported generalized aches and pains or the upper limb pain syndrome previously known as repetitive strain injury, in addition to arthritis, fibromyalgia and the hypermobility syndrome.

Tubiana (Tubiana and Chamagne 1993), a highly respected hand surgeon in France, reported that among 234 pianists, 52 suffered from the overuse syndrome, 43 the results of trauma, 21 had tendonitis, 88 had dystonia and 25 had problems which could be attributed to technical faults. Among 98 violinists, 33 had the overuse syndrome, 33 dystonia, 19 the results of trauma and 10 technical faults.

Lambert in his comprehensive review (Lambert 1992) reported that between 50% and 80% of musicians reported upper limb pain in the various published surveys. Fetter in 1993 confirmed that in all surveys published about two-thirds of an orchestra suffer aches and pains in the upper limb, and this was confirmed in his own study of the Baltimore Symphony Orchestra.

A recent survey of 55 orchestras worldwide carried out by the British Association of Performing Arts Medicine and the Féderation Internationale de Musique highlighted the physical, emotional and psychological problems faced by orchestral musicians. This material was presented at the First International Conference of Music Medicine held at York in April 1997. Over 1600 replies to a questionnaire were received. Twenty-seven per cent reported upper limb pain more than once a week, 16% suffered performance anxiety more than once a week and 70% reported performance anxiety during a performance. The top ten stresses reported were:

- conductors who sap your confidence
- incompetent conductors
- having problems with the instrument
- playing an orchestral solo
- illegible music, particularly music that had been photocopied several times in which quite often the ledger lines were lost: it might be difficult for people with failing eyesight to see this without leaning forward and getting chronic strain of the neck
- disorganized rehearsal time
- incompatible desk partners
- having medical problems that affected their work
- making a mistake when performing
- inadequate financial reward and worrying about finance in the event of illness.

There was a strong correlation between anxiety and upper limb pain, emphasizing again the way in which anxiety and worry cause muscle tension which results, in turn, in neck, shoulder and back pain. Forty-one per cent stated that sometimes their fingers were disobedient, and one wonders if this is an early sign of dystonia which can develop into the true clinical picture if there is no respite from chronic fatigue and excessive playing.

Very significantly 83% did not feel their training in school and conservatoires had prepared them for the stresses of being a musician. This emphasizes the vital role of music teachers, a role which to date too few have assumed in instruction in good posture, good practice technique and a sensible lifestyle in general.

A conductor present at the York conference defended his profession against the strictures reported in the questionnaire, pointing out that the conductor's role was to give precise guidance, to give clear directives, to explain the expectations being made and to create an intense relationship with musicians and be active in stress management. Unfortunately, too many conductors are not aware of their responsibilities to their musicians' health. This is to be deplored, for without an orchestra the conductor has no raison d'être. It must be accepted, of course, that the conductor himself has many stresses which he may inadvertently wish on the orchestra. He needs to know the music, the musicians, the management and the public, needing confidence, competence and credibility. The particular conductor accepted that conductors in general need better training and understanding of the orchestra's problems and better interpersonal skills.

The problems orchestras face with unsatisfactory acoustics was aired at the same conference. The Royal Festival Hall in London with its ultra-dry acoustics imposed problems on string players, particularly as they need more breathing time for their sound, thus making bowing harder work. The transition between good and bad acoustics in the same day – e.g. from the Royal Festival Hall to one of the recording studios – imposes its own problems.

Problems are also reported among music students. Manchester (Manchester 1988) reported on 246 music students who had had 8.5 episodes of performance-related upper limb problems per 100 musicians, with males being twice as commonly affected as females. An identifiable cause was established in 50%; the common causes were increase in playing time, change in

technique and change of repertoire. Of those with an identifiable cause, 41% had problems in the hand or wrist, 38% in the neck, 35% in the shoulder, 11% in the forearm and 10% in the elbow.

Hagglund (Hagglund 1996) reported on 137 music students, 61% of whom had upper limb symptoms which were attributed to long hours, excessive practice, technically demanding pieces and a change in technique.

Larsson (Larsson et al 1993) reported on 600 music students, of whom 50% had musculoskeletal symptoms during play. Of string players 77% reported symptoms, including loss of endurance in 25%, loss of facility in 18% and loss of strength in 18%. The commonly affected sites were the fingers, thumbs and shoulders. Again, they indicated that decreased playing time and a change in technique were most likely to relieve the symptoms.

Newmark and Lederman (Newmark and Lederman 1987) reported on a group of amateur orchestral musicians who usually played 1 hour a day, but went on a very intensive course for 1 week playing for 6–7 hours a day. Of these musicians, 72% developed new playing-related problems and 81%, who had significantly increased their practice, had marked symptoms.

In 1997 Winspur and Wynn Parry published their experiences with over 300 musicians. This experience now extends to over 600 musicians (Tables 1 and 2) attending a special performing arts medicine clinic. These clinics are part of the British Association of Performing Arts Medicine Trust's initiative. A telephone helpline has been

Table 1 Upper limb problems of musicians (n = 617)

Clear diagnosis	257	41%
Symptomatic hypermobility syndrome	17	10
True tenosynovitis	38	6
Rotator cuff/frozen shoulder	39	6
Old injury	68	9
Osteoarthritis	26	4
Thoracic outlet syndrome	14	2
Rheumatoid arthritis	8	
Low back pain	23	4
Ganglion	13	
Carpal tunnel syndrome	3	
Tennis elbow	8	
Technical causes		40%
Emotional/psychological causes		19%

Table 2 Diagnosis in 34 professional musicians undergoing hand surgery

Dupuytren's contracture	8	25%
Tumours (6 ganglions, 2 giant cell tumours)	8	25%
Trauma	7	20%
Carpal tunnel syndrome	5	15%
Osteoarthritis (arthrodesis)	3	
Cubital tunnel syndrome	2	
Osteoarthritis (synovectomy)	1	
	34	

established in central London which performing artists may consult. If it is felt that consultation with an experienced music medical practitioner is warranted, they are offered an appointment for a free consultation with a variety of specialists, including general physicians, rheumatologists, orthopaedic surgeons, hand surgeons, ENT surgeons and occupational physicians. In addition, there is a wide network of specialist instrumentalists who can advise on technique and performance practice. There is also access to highly experienced arts psychologists to discuss problems of stress, stage fright and performance anxiety. There is also a network of therapists to advise and treat patients with the full range of musculoskeletal problems, particularly physiotherapists, Alexander teachers and Feldenkreis experts. Most patients are referred by their general practitioners but many consult the helpline directly, either because they have difficulty in contacting their general practitioner or because the general practitioner has been unable to help.

Our series, we feel, is as near unselective as possible and represents the whole gamut of the problems experienced by musicians. We showed that only 41% of our patients had organic structural lesions, of which only 4% required surgery; 40% were regarded as suffering from technical problems in its widest sense; and 19% were suffering the effects of stress and anxiety but presenting with musculoskeletal symptoms.

Common conditions (see Chapter 7) in which there was a clear pathological diagnosis included cervical spondylosis, cervical ribs or thoracic outlet syndrome, clear-cut rotator cuff lesions, tennis or golfer's elbow, De Quervain's syndrome, trigger finger, osteoarthritis of the metacarpal

joints of the thumbs, painful ganglion, clear-cut carpal tunnel syndrome and tenosynovitis. Hypermobility was common and this is discussed as a separate issue as it is a most important finding in a musician with upper limb problems.

Medical evaluation of the musician

It is essential to examine the whole body in any musician complaining of upper limb pain. It is also important to examine them while playing. It is important to note the presence of deformities such as scoliosis, kyphosis, abnormal leg length,

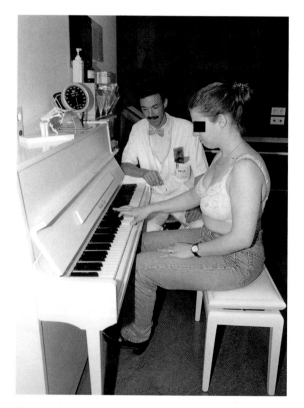

Figure 1

Well-equipped clinic for medical evaluation of musicians. Note the piano, and the fact that the musician is undressed (by courtesy of Dr ABM Rietveld).

lack of spinal mobility or stiffness of neck and shoulder (see Chapter 11). It should go without saying that, wherever possible, the musician should be observed with his instrument and should be stripped to make it possible to observe the posture and technique adopted (Fig. 1). Dr Rietveld in Holland has a piano in his clinic: in the case of non-transferable instruments, observation of the musician at work in his studio is often a revelation. It is not uncommon, for example, to find limitation of internal rotation of the shoulder in string players, which can seriously affect their performance. This may be as a result of an old rotator cuff lesion that has not responded to treatment or an incipient frozen shoulder. It is not uncommon for patients with proximal problems to present with symptoms distally. For example, a patient with a stiff and painful shoulder may alter the technique of fingering on a stringed instrument in order to relieve tension, and this in turn may lead to strain and fatigue of the distal muscles which may be the presenting symptom.

General medical conditions

The possibility of a general medical condition causing aches and pains must never be forgotten in young students who are overworking before auditions. The cause of their muscular fatigue may not be solely excess practice but may be an underlying symptom of early thyroid disease, diabetes or anaemia. In the established musician, alcohol abuse is not uncommon and should be tactfully and carefully sought. Fatigue and muscular pain may be the presenting symptoms of depression. Depressive illnesses are common in the general population. Musicians are no exception and their difficult lifestyle may precipitate or aggravate a depressive illness, and careful assessment of the possibility of depression and its treatment is vital. Antidepressant therapy can result in dramatic improvement in mood and attitude and its serotonin-sparing properties can often relieve chronic pain. Dystonia is discussed in detail at length in Chapter 14, but this is an important condition and should always be borne in mind. Patients present with painless inco-ordination, particularly in the early stages, and they should

be fully screened neurologically, so that a space-occupying lesion is not missed.

Technical problems

Examination of the musician with their instrument may immediately reveal that there is an inappropriate match of the musician's body to their instrument (see Chapter 3). We have seen cellists of small stature who have great problems in carrying their cello around and the provision of wheels (Fig. 2) has satisfactorily solved the problem of shoulder and arm pain. Patients with short arms may find the viola a difficult instrument. Very tall patients, that is patients over 5'11", may find the violin difficult because of the

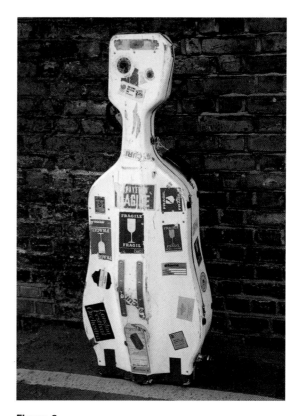

Figure 2

Cello case with wheels – to be pulled not carried.

large distance between the neck and the shoulder. An increased carrying angle of the elbow in a violinist may result in ulnar nerve irritation due to the prolonged flexion of the elbow required.

The general examination which is so important will have revealed whether there is any specific joint stiffness or weakness, e.g. after an old injury, a significant scoliosis or kyphosis, or an unsuspected mild congenital hemiplegia. All these conditions can lead to muscle fatigue and pain when holding the instrument. A judicious rehabilitation programme will restore function. The common causes of aches and pain due to technical problems are sometimes more subtle and require careful assessment of the musician playing for some time – it may require more than one visit, and a video taken of the musician playing which can be studied at leisure by both the physician and the patient is most useful. Not infrequently a musician will express amazement on seeing the technique actually adopted and will quickly appreciate how symptoms have arisen. The detection of hypermobility is extremely important. In the presence of marked hypermobility and relative weakness of the controlling muscles, muscular fatigue and pain are common: this can easily be remedied by intensive progressive rehabilitation programmes to build up both strength and stamina in the appropriate muscles (see Chapter 11).

Obviously, there are right and wrong ways of playing a musical instrument. Les Wright, a drummer in the Royal Air Force band, has told me that all apprentice drummers learn an exercise programme with the drumsticks to develop power and flexibility in the wrist which must be practised under supervision on a daily basis. He was unaware that any drummer ever had problems with painful wrists or hand in a full career in the band. Wajit Khan, the renowned sarod player, explained to me that painful wrists, hands or arms were rare in Indian string players. Most learn their skill from the earliest age. Wajit Khan comes from eight generations of players and playing is 'in the blood'. Constant practice with adequate breaks and slow gradual development of technique is the guard against problems. In fact backache from the posture required to be maintained for long periods is more of a problem. Therefore strict attention to good posture, balance and strength is all important. Similarly, tabla players have few problems with their hands, despite the mesmerizingly complex hand movements both in speed and rhythm they achieve. Again, it is years of progressive practice that prevents symptoms, but backache is a problem because of the prolonged straight sitting posture required.

Wrong ways involve excessive tension and inefficient use of muscles and joints which, in time, will lead to muscle fatigue and pain. This prompts alterations of technique and adjustments to avoid pain which may give rise to secondary complications, with strains of muscles and joints remote from the origin of the problem. For example, in a violinist abnormal tension in the shoulder muscles may lead to an attempt to relieve pain by excessive use of the wrist and fingers and the patient may then present with wrist and finger pain when the cause of the problem is to be sought further proximally.

Anything which creates excessive tension is unacceptable. Violinists should keep a reasonably straight bow, parallel with the bridge, and the wrist should not be too hyperflexed or rotated. Excessive extension of the wrist is likely to produce tension in the long flexors. The weight of the violin has to be taken either by the left hand or by the left collarbone and chin or equally by the two (Blum and Ahlers 1994). Most violinists prefer that the weight is taken at the chin, but it is essential that there is no tension between the neck and the shoulder. The lack of an adequate shoulder rest means the patient having to hunch the shoulder up and lean the neck too far forward, thus causing tension and spasm in the trapezius. Levy (Levy et al 1992) carried out electrical studies on the biceps, deltoid, trapezius and sternomastoid muscles of violinists while they played two musical selections. As neck dimensions increased, the shoulder rest was more likely to promote diminished electrical activity from the tested muscles and the investigators demonstrated that the shoulder rest had a great effect on muscles used to support the violin and that a proper rest may decrease susceptibility to musculoskeletal injury. Hunching of the right shoulder is also a potent cause of bad bowing technique, and spasm in these muscles provokes pain which may be both proximal and distal. Shoulder rests often only sit in one place and it is important to assess the efficiency of a shoulder rest carefully. String players with long necks, particularly those who are tall, may not be able to find a satisfactory rest commercially. William Benham, an Alexander teacher and a professional violinist, has designed special rests that are custom-made for patients with long necks and we have frequently been grateful to him for a custom-built rest which has completely solved the problem of shoulder and neck pain. An over-tight grip of the bow in all string players is a frequent cause of pain.

Joan Dixon, the doyenne of ergonomic problems in cellists, stated that there would be no upper limb pain if the cellist's movements were balanced, free and without tension. She emphasized the importance of a constant flow of arm movement with alternating relaxation and contraction. A tense forearm causes pain. Too tight a thumb grip causes pain along the extensor aspect of the thumb up to the elbow and even up to the shoulder. Many student cellists, she found, use extreme force all the time rather than only when it is necessary. She emphasized the importance of rotating the humerus as much as possible and not the forearm, because this gives a freer, stronger and more relaxed movement. A generally too-tensed, flexed posture over the cello leads to troublesome neck and back symptoms.

A great deal can be learnt by the music physician by looking at the general stance and approach to the instrument. Change of instrument and change of bow are a frequent cause of problems. Often for years the musician has learned to use a particular instrument in a particular way and a change in its shape, dimensions or tension means that the whole system has to be recoded, which can cause subtle changes in muscle joint dynamics and result in fatigue and pain.

Keyboard players are prone to various problems. The classical disorder is when the pianist plays with extended wrists instead of relaxed wrists and this causes marked strain on the extensor expansion. A crouched position over the piano leads to shoulder and neck pain.

Sakai (Sakai 1992) reviewed 40 Japanese pianists with hand and forearm pains as a result of overuse. The causes included tennis elbow, golfer's elbow, muscular pain in the forearm, pain in the flexor carpi radialis or ulnaris tendons, pain in the extensor retinaculum, De Quervain's tenosynovitis and pain in the thenar and hypothenar muscles. Of these pianists 30

attributed their problems to practising special keyboard techniques such as octaves, chords and fortissimo passages. These three common techniques accounted for a total of 77% of the problems. They noted that abduction of the thumb and fourth or fifth finger were responsible for many of the symptoms. Appropriate alteration of technique and building up muscle power was helpful in many cases. However, they point out that some pianists' hands, particularly young, small stature, female Japanese hands, are really too small for the demands placed upon them and the condition may not be curable.

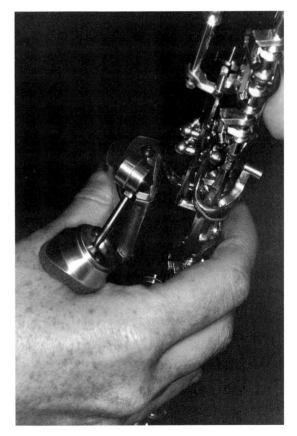

Figure 3

Adjustable 'Kooiman' thumb rest on an oboe adjusted such that most of the weight is transmitted directly on to the head of the metacarpal and not across the metaphalangeal or interphalangeal joints via a long moment arm (by courtesy of Howarth of London).

Woodwind instruments often cause problems. The static loading of the web space is common between the thumb and the index finger when supporting a clarinet or oboe, and playing the flute places weight on the digital nerve of the radial side of the left index finger and can often cause paraesthesias. There are now a whole variety of supports and straps and harnesses designed to take the pressure off the supporting structures and the musician should be urged to shop around to find the correct support for his particular problem (Fig. 3).

References

Blum J, Ahlers J (1994) Ergonomic considerations in violists' left shoulder pain. *Med Probl Perform Artists* **9**:1.

Critchley M, Henson RA, eds. (1977) Music and the brain: studies in the neurology of music. Charles C Thomas: Springfield, Ill.

Fetter BN (1993) Life in the orchestra. *Md Med J* **42**: 289–92.

Fishbein M, Middlestadt SE, Ottati V, Strauss S, Ellis A (1988) Medical problems among ICSOM musicians: overview of a national survey. *Med Probl Perform Artists* **3**:1–8.

Graffman G (1986) Doctor can you lend an ear? *Med Probl Perform Artists* **1**:3–4.

Hagglund KL (1996) A comparison of the physical and mental practices of music students. *Med Probl Perform Artists* **11**:99–107.

Lambert CM (1992) Hand and upper limb problems of instrumental musicians. *Br J Rheumatol* **31**:265–71.

Larsson L-G, Baum J, Mudholkar GS et al (1993) Nature and impact of musculoskeletal problems in a population of musicians. *Med Probl Perform Artists* **8**:73–6.

Levy CE, Lee WA, Brandfonberner AG et al (1992) Electromyographic analysis of muscular activity in the upper extremity generated by supporting a violin with and without a shoulder rest. *Med Probl Perform Artists* **7**:103–9.

Manchester RA (1988) The incidence of hand problems in music students. *Med Probl Perform Artists* **3**:15–18.

Newmark J, Lederman RJ (1987) Practice doesn't necessarily make perfect. Incidence of overuse syndromes in amateur instrumentalists. *Med Probl Perform Artists* **2**:93–7.

Sakai N (1992) Hand pain related to keyboard technique in pianists. *Med Probl Perform Artists* **7**:2.

Tubiana R, Chamagne P (1993) Les affections profesionelles du membre supérior chez les musiciens. *Bull Acad Natl Med* **177**:203–16.

Winspur I, Wynn Parry CB (1997) The musician's hand. *J Hand Surg* **22B**:433–40.

3
The interface

Introduction

Christopher B Wynn Parry

Many problems can arise as a result of a mismatch between the player and the instrument – the so-called interface (Markison 1990). The player's anatomy may not be suitable for the particular instrument. A harpist may not have sufficient reach to play the distant strings. The violist's arm may be too short to curve round a large viola. The violinist may have too long a neck for placing the instrument comfortably between chin and neck. A pianist may have too marked a lumbar lordosis to allow easy forward playing. A cellist or bassist may be too small or too slight easily to transport the instrument comfortably. The pianist's hands may be too small for easy playing of octaves. Anatomical anomalies such as a cervical rib or scalenus band may cause pressure on the plexus or vessels at the root of the neck from a stringed instrument. Hypermobility without strong muscles across the affected joints makes for vulnerability to strains and stresses. An increased carrying angle may cause irritation of the ulnar nerve at the elbow with stringed instruments.

Restriction of full range of movements of joints or weak muscles due to old trauma, particularly following inadequate rehabilitation, can seriously affect performance. Restriction of internal rotation of the shoulder seriously impairs bowing, as does weakness of (when winging) the scapula after, for example, neuralgic amyotrophy. Limited pronation affects ability to execute

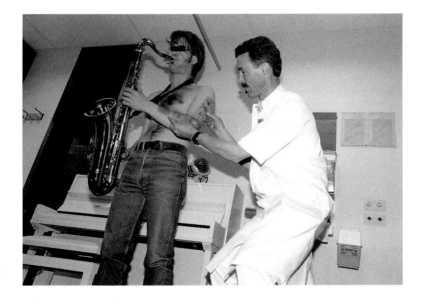

Figure 1

Careful assessment of the locomotor system *in toto* with the patient undressed (by courtesy of Dr ABM Rietveld).

chords on the piano and weak intrinsics in thumb musculature affect vibrato on stringed instruments and the support of wind instruments. Careful assessment of the locomotor system *in toto* in the undressed patient (Fig. 1) is needed to spot limited range of all upper limb joints and spine, presence of scoliosis, kyphosis, lordosis, disturbed scapulohumeral rhythm from old rotator cuff lesions, tightness of upper thoracic spine (a potent cause of aching and disordered technique in all types of instrumentalists), slight weakness globally in hitherto undetected congenital hemiplegia or birth injury.

Every musician should be screened for hypermobility of neck, shoulders, elbows, wrists, fingers, thumbs, spine and knees. Hypermobility is an important cause of general and local muscular symptoms (see Chapter 7). Clearly it is important to note other activities in the musician's life that may have caused problems or aggravated them, e.g. gardening, sport, typing. One of our patients developed pain in the thumbs from low bicycle handle bars, and previous traumas, particularly whiplash injuries, are a potent cause of neck and shoulder discomfort. Antecedent trauma may precipitate dystonia (see Chapter 14). Finally, a careful history related to the particular instrument must be taken:

- Has there been a recent change in the instrument? (Alternating between lute and guitar with their different neck dimensions can cause problems as the player has to recode for each one.)
- Is the new instrument different in size or weight?
- Does the new instrument require more effort, e.g. four-string as against five-string guitar, different tension of strings or a stiffness of action in a new piano?
- Has the style of playing changed?
- Has the repertory changed?
- Have new techniques been attempted? An attempt to incorporate a changed harpsichord fingering technique led to temporary dystonia in one front rank player.

Obviously wherever possible the musician should be observed playing the instrument, if necessary a video taken and a tape made with a running commentary as to when the pain starts. A visit to the rehearsal room or studio or obser-

vation in performance are all ideal. An observation at the end as well as at the beginning of a practice session can be revealing.

Finally, an assessment of general fitness should be made, both strength and stamina of muscles and cardiovascular function. One needs to be physically fit not only to cope with the instrument itself, particularly if it is cumbersome or heavy, but to withstand the rigours of practice, concerts, recording, teaching, travel and tours. Too few students are advised on these points and the opportunity should be taken in the clinic to deliver a short homily on fitness for music-making.

Woodwind

Christopher B Wynn Parry

The flute is somewhat of a devil for musculoskeletal problems; the left hand has to be held with the index metaphalangeal (MP) joint hyperextended to support the weight of the instrument. The flute is held below the level of the shoulder to avoid tension in the shoulders and neck and the left forearm from the strain of holding the instrument horizontally (Fig. 2). However, this means that the hand has to be tilted down to the right and in turn can strain the right neck muscles. Norris (1993) has designed an angled head joint, which allows the head to remain almost in the neutral position and allows also the right shoulder to be relaxed down. He points out that the right thumb is used to support the weight of the flute to provide opposition for the fingers as they press down on the keys and to stabilize the flute while playing notes in open position. The flute tends to be unstable due to the offset position of the rods on which the keys pivot, and may tend to roll in. This can be prevented by increasing the pressure between the flute and the chin while squeezing the flute between thumb and little finger of the right hand causing tension. The Bopep thumb support transforms the base of the flute from a convex to a concave surface and increases the distribution forces over a wider area of the thumb. But Norris finds that the flute still rolls in in open positions and so he devised a steady rest. This uses a non-slip cork-lined

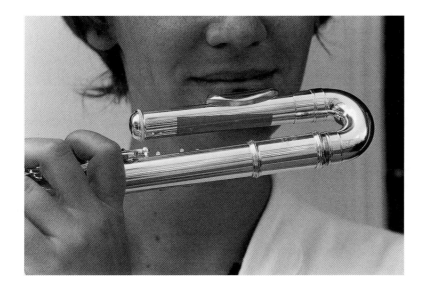

Figure 2

Curved mouthpiece on a flute to lower and reduce tension in the shoulders and neck and to reduce the stretch for shorter arms (by courtesy of All Flutes Plus, London).

metal clip which grips the flute and has an adjustable foam-padded metal extension custom-fitted to the thumb, thus distributing the pressure wider and distributing the weight of the rods through the base of the support preventing it from rolling inwards. Left-hand compression of the digital nerve of the index is not uncommon due to the hyperextended position of the finger and its role in supporting the flute by the ledge so-formed. Norris uses a foam-padded hook curling round the base of the left index finger, which relieves the tension and provides stability, but other types of device are available (Fig. 3).

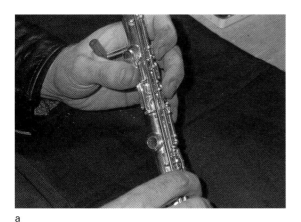

a

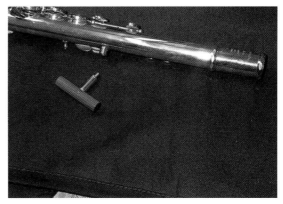

b

Figure 3

(a, b) Flute support to ease pressure on the radial digital nerve in the index finger and allow repositioning of the index MP joint (by courtesy of All Flutes Plus, London).

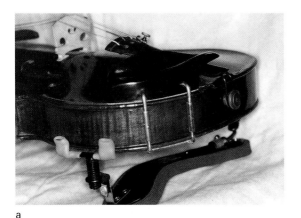
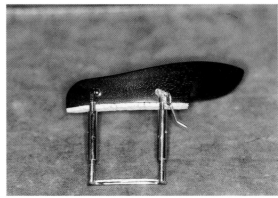

a   b

Figure 4

(a, b) Adjustable shoulder and chin support for violinists with longer necks (by courtesy of JP Guiver & Co., London).

Violin

The commonest problem in violin-playing is the tendency to hunch the left shoulder and push it forward, which not only causes fatigue in the trapezius and shoulder muscles, but in time leads to pain in the left arm and hand. Shoulder and chin rests are the standard means of overcoming this tendency, the hunch of the shoulder or leaning into the violin with the neck. Violinists with long necks are notoriously prone to upper limb problems owing to the difficulty in bridging the gap between chin and clavicular area (Fig. 4). Violinists must experiment until they find exactly the correct fit. In very tall individuals a suitable commercial rest may not be available. Then a custom-built rest should be prescribed. Benham, a violinist and Alexander teacher, has described such rests. In our clinic we have seen dramatic reduction in symptoms once a satisfactory custom-made rest has been provided. Excessive extension of the left wrist causes excessive tension in the flexors of the fingers and wrist. Similarly, excessive medial swinging of the elbow causes tension in the wrist and fingers. Unacceptable muscle tension in the right arm can be produced by failure to keep a straight bow parallel to the bridge. Hunching of the right shoulder when bowing will cause spasm and pain in the shoulder and neck muscles.

A common fault in all string players in the early stages of their career is the tendency to grip the bow too tightly, causing pain in the thumb and later pain in the origins of the extensor and flexors of wrist and fingers. In the following section Simon Fischer emphasizes strongly the need for balance in all parts of both arms. Good bowing technique in all stringed instruments demands full and free use of the arm. Restricted arc of movement causes a restricted and mean sound and inevitably results in tension and pain in the arm.

Technique and ease in violin-playing

Simon Fischer

Many players suffer the frustration of knowing that their playing could be better, easier or more comfortable, but without knowing how to go about improving it. Some go round in circles for decades without ever finding the answers to their questions, simply trying to survive from day to day or performance to performance.

When violinists feel restricted by tension in their arms, hands and fingers, there are usually a multitude of interrelated factors responsible. Many of these factors are subtle or invisible aspects of technique which, though seemingly insignificant, each set off a chain-reaction of tension that spreads throughout the entire playing. There are likely to be many separate chain-reactions all occurring at the same time, starting from different areas and reinforcing each other in a complex network.

In most cases, each of these subtle aspects of technique that produce tension are more a matter of technique needing to be improved, rather than it being the case that the technique is good but that unfortunately there is a lot of unexplainable tension.

Violin technique is a mosaic of 'techniques'. Five different notes on a keyboard instrument may require five virtually identical methods of depressing the keys. On the violin the same five notes may require five completely different methods of producing each note: the first note may require the bow to be placed on the string silently, then to move along the string with a bow speed that changes from fast to slow and a pressure that changes from heavy to light; the second note may be played by dropping a finger on to the string without affecting the motion of the bow at all; the next note may require the bow to pivot across to another string at the same time as changing direction, coupled with a movement of the left hand to another area of the fingerboard; and so on.

Whether you are an elementary or a concert violinist, playing the easiest or the most difficult piece, most of the techniques used are the same. Apart from certain virtuoso elements that do not arise in simpler playing, to an extent an 'easy' piece is one where few different techniques have to be employed at the same time or in close succession; a 'difficult' piece is one where there may be dozens of different techniques employed simultaneously or in extremely rapid sequence.

The world-famous violin teacher Dorothy DeLay once said: 'Sometimes I wonder why anybody is ever interested in anything I have to say – it all seems so simple!' The sort of playing she is typically dealing with, i.e. the big concertos and technical show-pieces, is made up of the same 'basics' that elementary pieces are. A concerto may be a thousand times more difficult than an elementary piece, but the language used to describe what is happening in them is basically the same for both.

The mechanics of playing are not intangible like the musical-expressive side of playing. 'Artistry', 'musicality', 'expression', 'communication', 'talent' and suchlike are aspects of a veiled world which cannot easily be quantified and defined. But the entire physical side of playing – the concrete reality of the hands and the bow and the string and how they work – is fully describable from beginning to end, and therefore teachable or changeable.

The key that opens the door to every aspect of technique on a string instrument is thinking in terms of proportions. 'Divine proportionality', as Leonardo di Vinci called it, is also the fundamental basis of every musical consideration: dynamics, intonation, tempo, and so on.

The moment you begin to consider your playing in terms of the proportions of one movement (or aspect of playing) to another, the flood gates open and you can find that, far from not knowing how to proceed in solving problems of technique and/or tension, you have a non-stop stream of information always available and can work on yourself as potently as any teacher can work on you.

Each element or facet of playing, musical or technical, can be expressed in terms of proportions. Everything is always a question of measurement: how fast the finger drops or lifts relative to the tempo; how fast the bow moves relative to the pressure and distance from the bridge; different speeds and widths in the vibrato; different heights and lengths in the spiccato, and so on. The position of the violin, and the placement of the hands and fingers on the instrument and bow, are also questions of proportions touched upon in the following pages.

Paradigms

Practice has little to do with training muscles. The muscles are always innocent, simply carrying out instructions from the brain. Playing is literally 'all in the mind'. Suppose you sight-read through a piece, making many mistakes of intonation, sound, rhythm and so on. Then you practise it for 2 hours, after which you can play it fluently. What has changed? Physically you have not changed at all. It is not like building up in a gym for a month, after which the muscles you have trained are now physically different. All that has changed is that your mental picture, of what and how to play, has now taken shape. The same applies to building, shaping or redesigning technique: it is not the strength or the state of the muscle, but the thought behind the muscle, that counts.

If you want to change the way you play, you have to change the way you think about your playing. One of the chief jobs of the teacher is not only to present and implement helpful ideas, but also to weed out the unhelpful ideas that are getting in the way. The problem is that many of these may be buried so deeply that, although they continue to exert an influence, they are forever hidden and forgotten whatever the good intentions of the teacher or the student.

One of my first pupils was a boy of 9 who, in 3 years, developed from a poor Grade 1 standard into a poor Grade 5 standard. He always had a very 'wooden' bow arm and was never able to find that sensuous quality of bowing that distinguishes a natural string player. We worked on his bowing constantly with no real improvement, except that as the years went by he was able to play harder pieces – but still with the wooden tone and tension.

Finally a new fragment of thought came up which explained why progress had been so limited. *He had always thought that the bow moved in a straight line*. In fact there is no bow stroke on the violin that moves in a straight line: every stroke is curved, or moving in a slight arc, the bow playing (even if imperceptibly) *around* the string.

Perhaps the very first time he saw a violin being played he unconsciously registered the impression of the bow moving in a straight line as a fact. Or perhaps his first teachers, in trying to get him to draw the bow parallel with the bridge, had unwittingly communicated the idea of a straight line. Wherever it had come from, this single erroneous idea, active but hidden at the back of his mind, short-circuited his every effort to play.

If I want to demonstrate symptoms of tension and awkwardness in bowing, all I need do is try to draw the bow in a 'straight line': the symptoms appear at once with startling naturalness. With sufficient will-power and determination many players can reach quite a high standard even with such an in-built deficiency as trying to play in a straight line – but there will always be an element of strain or 'something not quite right' about their playing.

A new student coming for a lesson recently had an awkward-looking left-hand action. I made various suggestions which she was slow to pick up. She began to seem rather untalented. Then it came out that she had always thought no finger should ever touch another finger. This explained not only her original awkwardness but also her slowness at finding any new feeling: she was trying to fulfil the paradigm of fingers not touching each other while at the same time trying to fulfil my suggestions.

Tone production is an area where a change of concept can work wonders in bringing relaxation and ease into the right hand and arm. Remarkably few string players have a clear understanding of what the hair of the bow actually does to the string, and how sound is the result of certain proportions of speed of bow and pressure relative to the distance from the bridge. This is not to say that they cannot play with a beautiful tone – a good player with a natural feel for the string, playing with inspiration, does not require an intellectual understanding in order to play; nevertheless, most players do find enormous benefits of increased control and security when they start to work on their tone in a systematic way using carefully weighed proportions of speed and pressure at different distances from the bridge.

Another important aspect is the concept of release. There must be as many releases of the muscles as there are contractions. A useful analogy is the binary code used in computers, where all information is reduced to numbers made up of ones and zeros – either 'on' or 'off'. Similarly, the actions of the left hand could be expressed as a string of digits, '1' representing a muscle in use (i.e. contracted) and '0' representing the same muscle released.

In some passages the sequence would be '10101010', i.e. every action immediately followed by a release before another action. In other passages it would be more a matter of releasing *often enough*, as in '10111011110'. But if the number reads '11111111' for too long, tension is inevitable. Discovering where to release – or more than that, beginning to approach every action on the violin from the standpoint of constant release and 'not-doing' – is often a major, defining step that can quickly help a player develop greater ease.

Difference between conscious control and autonomic

The degree to which individuals are able to let go of conscious control when they are making music, to *let* the arms, hands and fingers function without interference, can define the level of musical and technical achievement they are able to attain. It is not possible to play a musical instrument as complex and subtle as the violin using conscious control, but our bodies are clever enough to play it themselves. The autonomic nervous system is a super-computer which responds at lightning speed to the musical images we hold in our mind, producing a quickness, smoothness and flow of muscular action that we can only parody using conscious control.

A simple experiment: most people can whistle a note and then sing exactly the same note, then the same a tone higher, and so on. To be able to shape the vocal chords or the lips to within hundredths of a millimetre is a miraculous ability that we cannot take much credit for, since we could not possibly do it 'ourselves' using conscious control.

The great pianist Artur Schnabel said that the player has to be 100% the 'inner man', and 100% the 'outer man', at the same time. While remaining in overall conscious control of the playing, and occasionally even making deliberate technical judgements note by note, at the same time we must simply focus on the musical drama and expression and let our bodies perform all that is necessary to produce the musical result we picture.

During any 1 second of playing the brain sends thousands of messages to the muscles in the fingers holding the bow (for instance). The player could only send one or two conscious messages in the same period of time. All the player can do is hold the bow in such a way that he does not in any way inhibit the tiny adjustments to the bow hand that the autonomic nervous system commands. The player must concentrate on the music, and if the technical defaults are correct the right physical responses will follow.

On the physical plane, effort rewards. If I am hammering a nail, the harder and the faster I hit it the sooner the job is done. On the mental or emotional planes, the reverse is true: effort defeats. It is the harder you do *not* try, the easier everything becomes. The TV commentary during the 1997 tennis quarterfinal at Wimbledon in which Michael Stich soundly defeated the British champion Tim Henman made the parallels between sport and violin playing obvious. Henman had been playing very well in the matches preceding this one and his tennis was full of neat, clever or daring shots that won him point after point. In this match, he was still making those same shots but they were all played long or wide and missed repeatedly. At one point the commentator remarked: 'Tim Henman is trying too hard. When you are trying as hard as he is, all the playing goes on to a conscious level, instead of remaining on a deep, instinctive level. He needs to forget himself. He should just run to the ball and hit it, and remember what it feels like to *enjoy* hitting the ball, *without caring so much about the result*.'

Mental rehearsal

Mental rehearsal means visualizing exactly how you want to play the beginning, middle and end of each note and phrase, as well as the physical actions that produce them, as clearly as if you were watching an internal video. A mere 'wish' or optimistic attitude is not enough: the pictures need to be in great detail and include precise physical motions, the musical drama and expression, tonal colours, general ease of playing, and so on.

What is fascinating about mental rehearsal is that in your mind's eye you see exactly the same strengths and weaknesses as exist in your actual playing. For example, if your hand habitually goes tight when you play a particular note or phrase, you will see yourself tensing when you imagine playing. This is because you are accessing directly the very same 'computer program' that 'runs' your playing. By changing the images in your mind, the next time you pick up the instrument you find your playing has changed too.

All the most successful performers in any field rehearse mentally, whether they have a name for it and do it knowingly and deliberately or not. They relish every opportunity to run their performance through the mind in a constant process of sculpting and refining the vision – on trains, in the bath, in bed, while walking down the street. This is why players nearing a performance may often seem slightly distant and distracted, and require solitude and isolation.

Why are violin or viola players so at risk of tension?

1. Perhaps the first inherent problem is the way the left hand has to be placed on the neck of the violin. Only the violin and the viola require that the player rotate the left forearm clockwise (in order that the fingers can reach the strings) in such an unusual fashion. By comparison, every other orchestral instrument requires a much more natural position of the arms and hands. The further the violin is pointed in front of the player, the greater the clockwise rotation of the forearm. If the hand is positioned correctly on the instrument, and the instrument is held at the best angle to the body, it is possible to play with great ease. Tension in the wrist and hand is likely if the violin is pointed unnecessarily far in front, and if the hand is twisted excessively clockwise.

2. Another inherent problem is the way the instrument is positioned between the collarbone and the chin. Trying to hold the violin by pressing down with the chin (while at the same time pushing up with the shoulder) is an all-too-easy trap to fall into. If the neck is tense or fixed in a state of imbalance, tension soon spreads to the shoulders and from there to the arms and back. Keeping the neck free is one of the central tenets of the Alexander technique. If the neck is not free, this alone is sufficient to prevent the rest of the system from operating in a state of balance, continual release and easy movement.

3. The fingers must press the strings down with great subtlety and sensitivity, using the minimum finger pressure possible (just enough to stop the string enough to make a proper sound). Very often, the string does not even have to be pressed down far enough to touch the fingerboard. Excessive finger pressure has the effect of locking the hand into a vice-like grip on the neck of the instrument. It necessitates proportionate counterpressure from the thumb, the opposing fingers and thumb working in a vicious circle towards less and less ease of movement.

There are other factors which can cause tension, many of which will be touched upon below. But taking just these three examples alone, it is easy to see how problems can arise. Picture the violinist who plays with the scroll of the violin too far in front, twisting the left forearm uncomfortably clockwise, pressing the chin into the chin rest hard enough to cause sores and abscesses on the neck and tension in the shoulders and back, pressing the fingers into the strings hard enough to cause calluses on the fingertips . . . and sustaining all this for many hours each day.

Principal areas of potential difficulty

The following list includes the most common technical areas where tension typically arises. Most players would recognize at least a few items on the list as applying to themselves. There are many to whom only a few items would *not* apply.

- *Basic posture*. The violinist who has no postural deficiencies is rare. Typical areas of concern for violinists of all ages, standards and branches of the music profession are:
  - There must be sufficient 'grounding', the weight of the body naturally feeding down into the floor or the sitting bones.
  - The hip joint must not collapse forwards, a condition noticeable in many violinists.
  - The player must not 'pull down', bending forward in the region of the diaphragm, which causes the upper back to bend forward and the shoulders to pull in.

- The head must always be in a state of balance – not held in a fixed position – on top of the spine.
- *Angle of the violin to the player.* Many players use an angle of the instrument inappropriate to the length of their arms. Long arms: the violin should be held more to the left. Short arms: the violin should be held more to the right.
- *Angle of the violin to the floor.* Other specific problems are caused by holding the scroll too low, so that the instrument slopes down towards the floor.
- *Tilt of violin.* If the violin is too tilted clockwise along its axis, the top string does not give enough support to the bow, causing weak tone production. If the violin is too flat, playing on the lowest string becomes unnecessarily effortful.
- *Position of chin rest on instrument.* Long-armed players with the chin too much in the centre of the violin may lose some of the activity of the right upper arm. Short-armed players with the chin too far to the left of the violin may find it impossible to reach the end of the bow without strain in the bow arm.
- *Correct placement of chin on chin rest.* The difference between correct and incorrect placing of the chin on the chin rest may seem to slight as to be insignificant, yet the difference in results can be enormous.
- *Placement of hand on the neck of the violin.* Cases of players with small hands positioned too low in relation to the fingerboard are rare, but there are always frequent examples of players with large hands positioned too high.
- *Angle of base knuckle joints to fingerboard.* The angle is largely determined by which part of the fingertip contacts the string. The more the finger is placed on the far side of the fingertip (the side closest to the thumb), the more angled up are the knuckles; the more the finger is placed on the near side of the fingertip, the more the knuckles are parallel with the fingerboard.
- *Wrong part of the fingertip leading to wrong angle of base joints and elbow.* Which part of the fingertip contacts the string is one of the most crucial issues because it affects several other areas directly.
- *Concept of thumb.* For many players, this can be another case of the cure lying in the realization. Once they have understood that the thumb is actually the longest, not the shortest, finger on the hand and that, in effect, it has the same number of phalanxes as the other fingers, a natural release is likely to develop over time.
- *Squeezing the thumb next to the first finger.* Keeping an open space between the middle joint of the left thumb and the very base of the index finger is vitally important, since any squeezing immediately locks the hand.
- *Basing the left hand position on the upper more than the lower finger.* Most players would benefit from addressing this interesting and difficult-to-correct area.
- *Moving fingers from the base joint.* The main movement of the left fingers must be from the base joints, the rest of the hand remaining entirely still.
- *Finger pressure.* Throughout nearly all playing the correct amount of finger pressure is *as much as necessary (to stop the string properly) but as little as possible.* After the initial impact the finger releases the string slightly. The default should be 'drop-release' rather than 'drop-press'. Excessive finger pressure is one of the single most common, and at the same time most damaging, problem areas of technique.
- *Squeezing fingers together.* Since every hand is different the amount of space between the fingers varies from player to player. Some hands naturally have considerable space between fingers in most situations of playing, while other hands may find the fingers constantly touching each other. The key element is for there to be no *active sideways pressing* against another finger as part of stopping a note. Which part of the fingertip touches the string is one of the main factors determining how much space there is between the fingers.
- *Height of fingers.* The faster the passage the nearer the fingers must stay to the strings. Raising the fingers too high doubles or triples the energy used for the passage and can make fast playing impossible. An orchestral player with a too-high finger action, spending 6 hours a day playing furiously fast and difficult symphonic music, runs the risk of extreme fatigue.
- *Vibrato mechanism.* Of all the many issues concerning vibrato, the most common difficulties arise from the following:

- There should be only one active direction of movement in vibrato: *forward* to the in-tune note.
- Finger pressure should be heavier during the forward movement, lighter during the backward movement.
- *Left wrist.* In low positions the ideal is for the left forearm and the back of the hand to be in a straight line continuing up to the middle joint of the fingers. The wrist should quickly return to its normal position in a state of release.
- *Left upper arm.* The best position of the elbow is *only as far to the right as necessary (for the fingers to reach the strings), and no further.*
- *The left shoulder.* Except for those players with very short necks the violin alone is often not sufficient to fill the space between the collarbone and the chin. Raising the left shoulder to fill the gap, holding it in a state of ever-accumulating tension, is very common even amongst the highest-standard players. A permanently raised shoulder causes left upper arm tension, as well as the tendency to counterpress with the chin.
- *Placement of the right thumb on the bow.* The thumb should be placed diagonally with the left side of the thumb (as seen from the player's point of view when the thumb is in position) touching the wood of the bow and the right side of the thumb against the shaped thumb-piece on the bow. The amount of counterpressure should always be as much as necessary but as little as possible.
- *Bow hold: first finger position in relation to the thumb.* An efficient bow hold places the second finger almost opposite the thumb but positioned ever-so-slightly to the left of centre (as seen from the player's viewpoint), with the first finger correspondingly further away from the thumb.
- *Wrong position of the little finger on bow.* The role of the little finger is to balance the weight of the bow, particularly in the lower half of the bow but also in the upper half.
- *Tilt of bow.* The tilt of the bow (i.e. whether the side of the hair, or the flat of the hair, contacts the string), is an issue that many players neglect to consider. Using flat hair can give twice the tone for half the effort.
- *Forearm rotation.* The vertical movement of the upper arm is the main part of the arm used to cross from one string to another, but the hand and forearm can also take part.
- *Localizing all actions.* This means doing only the minimum that is required to perform the left or right hand action, and nothing else. The action takes place in one locality, without all sorts of unnecessary simultaneous actions happening elsewhere.

One of the starting points for improvement is the rigorous study of technique in minutiae. In almost every example of a player suffering from debilitating tension there are simple technical/physical causes that can quickly be rectified. It really is never too late, and players of any age and stage can continue to polish and refine their overall technique and move ever closer to truly effortless playing.

Guitar

Christopher B Wynn Parry with John Williams

John Williams, the world-famous guitarist, talked about and demonstrated to me over several hours the principles of correct guitar technique to avoid muscular problems and to produce the best sound. He pays tribute to his father, who was a famous classical guitarist and teacher in Australia and England and brought him up from the earliest days in the correct approach to playing. He went about playing the guitar in the same way as behaviour in everyday life, aiming to relax as much as possible and use minimal energy to gain the desired effect.

All techniques are contrived and basically unnatural for the guitar; there is an underlying conflict between technique and natural behaviour. For example, scales are natural, thirds unnatural. The hand moves up and down in a natural, physiological manner when strumming; as the finger is moving up and down on the same string, which is a natural movement; but when the fingers work alternately in the same direction, the movement already has become artificial. In order for the right hand to move freely across and up and down the strings for different tone colours and dynamics, and for the left hand to reach to all parts of the fingerboard comfortably, particularly the high part of

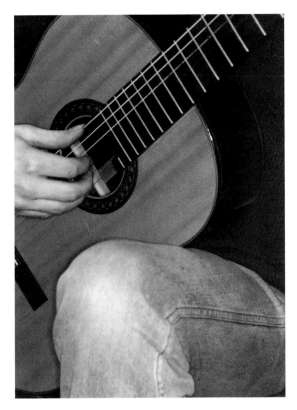

Figure 5

Raised position of the left foot to bring the guitar into comfortable range.

The technique of finger movement is very small and localized. As Simon Fischer points out, for every effect there is a cause and the cause of an unnatural postural position must be found. There is often a psychological background which must be sought. In the Renaissance, single note playing took place with thumb and finger, not index and middle, so the thumb down and finger up incorporates a natural rhythm. Classical technique has no natural rhythm. It is good for control and evenness of sound, but the static position of the wrist is unnatural, with movement occurring almost entirely at the proximal interphalangeal (PIP) joint with some slight movement of the distal interphalangeal (DIP) joint and least of all at the MP joint. Contrary to the case when playing piano or violin, very little movement is involved either in the upper limb or in the body as a whole.

The relaxed position with the guitar is as much a psychological as a technical approach. John Williams was an only child and used to sit back with his arms clasped, elbows bent and shoulders and neck hunched forward to catch the adults' conversation. His father asked him why he sat so, and the answer was that he was listening; but his father explained that it was a negative and tense withdrawal posture. Even now, when John finds himself in this position on a social occasion, he quickly corrects it and relaxes into a more physiological position.

John attributes his lack of muscular problems in his career to early upbringing and instillation of correct relaxed psychological and physical approach. Most guitarists place their left foot on a footstool, though some use a cushion on the left knee instead. There is inevitably a slight twisting of the torso due to the instrument's dimensions. These factors make it all the more imperative to change position after short periods of practice or playing. John never practises for more than 30 minutes at a time. At the end of a practice spell he will put down the guitar and stretch his arms, neck and body, relieving the static stresses and moving to the opposite positions to those adopted in playing. He will walk around, look up a reference, have a cup of tea, make a short telephone call and then resume the instrument. He says it takes 4 hours to do 2½ hours' practice or 3 hours to do 1½ hours. In order to avoid strain, he avoids contrived plans of practice, e.g. 15 minutes playing scales, 15 minutes exercising, 2 hours on the music

the fingerboard, a sitting position is adopted with the left foot supported in order to bring the butt high enough to give a comfortable range (Fig. 5). Apart from movement of the fingers of the left hand along the strings, and to some extent the fingers of the right hand up and down the strings, there are no natural movements of the fingers, wrist and arm which are in a sense related to music in movement. This is contrary to the case in other instruments; for example in the violin the bow goes up and down, and in the piano the whole arm is moving, but there is very little movement for a guitarist. The position of the left hand is more comfortable for a violinist or cellist than for a guitarist. The way the right elbow rests on the large butt of the guitar is unrelated to the music and is static.

repeating difficult passages over and over again at the same mechanical speed, which can entrench what is incorrect and make matters worse. Practice-like playing should be varied and fun. If it is not, one should find ways of making it so. One does not have to go through 4 hours of hell every day. How much wisdom is contained in these words is clear when one realizes that most musicians' life is lived in practice. Physical and psychological problems in the main stem from bad practice techniques, lack of warm-up or cooling down, too-long sessions, unrelaxed frame of mind, fear of performance, lack of positive thinking. We discussed the question of general exercise regimes in sport. He believes that the co-ordination so necessary in playing the guitar will be reflected in competitive competence in games. He agrees that contact sport should be eschewed. He likes to walk and plays tennis and a lot of table tennis. Only if the weather is bad does he spend for up to 10 minutes on a static bicycle. His forebears, of course, in Renaissance times would have exercised and conversed in the long galleries. He feels strongly that teachers should emulate his father's approach. Because the guitar is unnatural, teaching may concentrate on more specific techniques and this may create more problems than solutions. John's father told him to imagine that the movement of his two fingers was like pedalling a bicycle; this in general is a more natural rhythm. Guitarists as well as pianists, wind players and string players, suffer from dystonia. The finger will flex but will not return. Another finger will extend at the same time. He knows of three leading guitarists with such problems and in one it has occurred early in his career (see Chapter 14).

The music stand is important. It differs in practice from that used in performance where it must be lower so the audience can see the player. The player of course has to look down, straining the neck and shoulders, and the projection of sound suffers.

Position is as follows. The left knee is held at just more than 90° (see Fig. 5); the hip is slightly more flexed than 90°, the foot flat; the right leg has to be out of the way. The curve of the instrument is on the left side and the butt rests lightly on the right side. The right elbow loosely holds the guitar in position, which presses well into the right chest but touches loosely on the left due to the body torsion required. There should be very little tension in the elbow muscles, particularly in quiet passages. The

left wrist is very slightly flexed but above the fifth position is extended. John's father emphasized the natural curve of the fingers coming down on the strings, to counteract the tendency to flex the wrist. Strength is from extended position and flexion therefore should be avoided.

Finally, when discussing performance anxiety, he stated that to him it was partly a sort of conceit. Nervousness is due to the belief that one has got to do the best always in order to preserve one's self-image and avoid adverse criticism. The right attitude is the joy of music-making and the delight in sharing it with one's listeners, never as an ego trip.

Cello

Joan Dixon, the doyenne of cello pedagogues, repeatedly stated that if movements are free and full, the posture balanced and no tension present in the neck or back, playing the cello should cause no problems at all. No group of muscles should ever be held in tension for more than a very short time. There should be a constant flow of movement with alternating relaxation and contraction. It should be possible to put a fist between the neck of the cello and the chest. A tight grip with the thumb on the bow causes pain in the thumb which in time spreads up to the elbow. Too many cellists, particularly students, use maximum force all the time, rather than only when necessary, thus inevitably over time developing painful wrists and elbows. Some cellists raise their shoulders for emotional effects and keep them raised for too long. Some encompass the cello as if it were about to disappear down the aisle, which results in neck, shoulder and back pain. As in all string playing, the aim is use of minimal energy and maximum flow of the arm. Humeral rather than radial ulnar rotation is preferred. This produces a stronger and freer movement and there is less tension on the elbow fixators.

Technique

Christopher B Wynn Parry with Bernard Gregor-Smith

We are grateful to Bernard Gregor-Smith, a noted soloist and the cellist of the world-famous

Lindsay Quartet, for the following comments. He has long been concerned with teaching the correct approach to the cello to avoid musculo-skeletal problems and to produce the finest sound.

General position

On sitting down to play the cello it is necessary first of all to know and understand the correct sitting position. A cellist needs to find a balanced position between a 'flop' position and an exaggerated one (supported muscularly or forced). An important factor to be borne in mind is the height of the chair seat, which should be related to the height of the player. The seat should be level (not sloping backwards, though a slight slope forwards is possible), and should not exceed the height of the knee.

This balanced position is the most natural for the spine, allowing maximum freedom to the ribcage and thus ensuring regular uncramped breathing, a point worth mentioning as a great deal of unwanted, hindering tension stems from the holding of the breath. It should feel natural for the torso to incline itself towards the cello, counteracting the tendency to be pushed back by the weight of the cello on the chest, a bad position which creates one of the most prevalent back problems in cellists. This learning forward should come from the base of the pelvis and not halfway up the spine, another cause of the inordinate number of back disorders of which cellists complain. A somewhat controversial point is that which concerns the height and angle of the cello in relation to the floor. Many cellists have experimented with 'end-pins', but if one maintains a balanced position, some variations are possible without creating physical stress.

We can picture the whole arm as a system of levers, each having its own axis and capable of moving in a plane different from the others. Hand and forearm are carried by the upper arm, and therefore the freedom of movement rests primarily with the upper arm. All these are set in motion by our muscles and it is interesting to observe that the muscles that move a joint always lie in the next highest joint. Strength and greatest freedom of movement lie together in the upper arm. Hence this wonderful mechanism has levers which move with varying degrees of freedom on different planes, permitting countless forms of movement. Understanding the workings of the bow arm helps us to gauge correctly the amount of exertion necessary and to avoid much which is unnecessary.

Right arm

The use of the right arm is the most difficult aspect of string playing, as a great deal of movement has to be combined with flexibility, relaxation and free weight of the arm. All differing techniques should be based on the natural laws of the arm to obtain good art. Weight in the arm in its many degrees should be used, not muscular force. This weight is increased or decreased by our shoulder muscles. A large, full tone needs more weight from the arm on the string, therefore our muscles release the arm the required amount. If we need a light stroke, as in pianissimo, then we suspend the arm, holding off its weight so that the arm has a feeling of being 'airborne'. Many problems in the arm and shoulder are caused by not observing these rules of prime importance. The most important element in playing, the right arm, is the real player: the paintbrush hand. When the weight is permanently suspended in fixed tension and muscular force fights this for greater tone, a cramped sound, inhibited freedom and a painful arm and shoulder result. This can lead to the 'worst scenario', the cementing of the upper arm to the shoulder, negating the freest joint we have and preventing any extended possibility for great expression with the bow.

Every part of the arm and hand is of equal importance, but the wrist is not the chief joint in the art of bowing. The wrist is only stiff if we hold the bow with stiff fingers or stiffened forearm; it is a joint or hinge, and is supple by nature. It is, in my opinion, a subordinate joint in the system of levers – its function is to mediate between the movements of the arm and those of the bow. It should smooth and polish otherwise awkward arm movements to perfect them. An overactive wrist destroys a large, sonorous tone, and causes a wobbly lack of contact in the bow change from one direction to another. This, too, causes the unfortunate player to use force and create an opposition of movements causing in time pain in the elbow and upper arm.

Rock guitar

Christopher B Wynn Parry with Jane Kember

Jane Kember, our specialist physiotherapist, has had long experience of treating rock guitarists (Kember 1995a–g). She finds that common problems are forearm and wrist pain, both during and after playing. She notices that poor posture is common and poor technique is a frequent cause of disability. She is particularly impressed by the effects of old trauma, especially whiplash injuries, on the development of symptoms. Shoulder and neck pains are common and she often notices a muscle imbalance around the shoulder girdle. She stresses the importance of the interface and the necessity of choosing the correct guitar. Where string length is concerned, the longer the string, the greater the distance between the frets and therefore the more stretch of fingers is needed.

Neck size varies from both thin, flat curve to a thick and flat and one must choose the appropriate size for the particular hand and finger size of the instrumentalist. The shape of the guitar should be chosen for comfortable playing and to fit the musician's own body. Too large a shape brings the right arm into a poor lifted playing posture or will tempt the player to suspend the guitar too low to enable the hand to get on the string. It is very important that guitars should be supported with a broad strap to help distribute the weight, and should not cause tension at the cervicothoracic junction. The vast majority of self-taught players have been given or bought instruments without any such ergonomic advice and these may be quite unsuitable for their body build.

Posture

Many students practise for long hours sitting slumped on a bed or cross-legged. Good seating or standing posture is vital to prevent poor neck, thoracic or lumbar curves. Pain may develop in the wrists and hands from playing for too long in a poor posture. A protracted scapula places the whole arm in an awkward position and this results in a stiffly held elbow with the wrist being held too flexed to maintain the playing position.

It is important that the shoulder should be fully mobile with a freely moving elbow to allow relaxed, balanced playing action. Advice on warm-ups, playing times and the position of the guitar are necessary and this may vary with each individual. Practice of difficult pieces should be split up and interspersed with easier music so that non-stop repetitive work will not trigger symptoms.

When treating a guitarist, a physiotherapist should always take the opportunity to discuss their general lifestyle and their approach to travel and transport. Unless the player belongs to a large professional group, there will be heavy carrying involved, with the various amplification equipments. Care with lifting amplifiers is necessary when setting up and loading into transport. Stress levels when performing are reduced if the band is well rehearsed and there is no rush when setting up and performing and the players have a good feel for the acoustic. They may find that alcohol and even drugs may seem to relax them and help their anxiety before performance and even the performance itself, but as is well recognized the long-term effects can be disastrous and players need to be counselled in the hope that this sort of problem can be averted. When they are on the road, travelling from one gig to another, eating and sleeping patterns are of course altered. It is most important to provide adequate breaks in the schedule so that chronic fatigue does not develop, and it is vital that they have regular and properly balanced meals.

Piano

Carola Grindea

If someone walked around with his left shoulder raised, his neck twisted to the left and tilted chin down and his left arm outstretched, palm outward, for 6–8 hours a day for years, he would assuredly develop marked and permanent postural deformities, even if he never played the violin.

Thus began Dr Earl Owen's article in an issue of the *Quarterly Magazine* of the New South Wales Music Teachers' Association. Similarly, pianists playing for many hours every day, for years, with incorrect posture, stiffness in the wrists, elbows, shoulders, forearms, upper arms and the neck and back, would certainly develop physical problems and marked psychological trauma.

Problems presented by keyboard players

The various physical injuries and medical problems I encounter at the International Society for the Study of Tension in Performance (ISSTIP) Performing Arts Clinic are dealt with by appropriate specialists. Psychological problems are referred to arts psychologist counsellors while I work with every musician who seeks our advice.

In my experience, most performance-related aches and pains seem to be caused by excessive tension, incorrect posture and positioning of the joints or incorrect ergonomics: the interaction between the player and the instrument. This results in interference with muscular co-ordination and the freedom of breathing. Once these imbalances are corrected, pain is usually abolished. Musicians must understand the cause or causes of their problems and then undertake a programme of retraining so that they know how to cope with their studies and practice and their career in general. I have devised a simple approach which requires between one and several sessions. This involves learning to liberate muscles of unnecessary tension, followed by studying a piano technique using natural movements only.

Causes of physical problems and injuries

Tension is essential for good performance, but it should be positive tension, which translates into an intensity created through the total involvement of the artist in his or her music-making. It is the negative aspect which is our concern, that which can be very destructive, causing much damage, both physical and psychological. In dealing with problems created by tension, we have to study muscular and nervous tension, and this is not easy. These two types of tension appear simultaneously and there is a continuous interplay between them; anxiety of the mind in any degree tends to cause rigidity in the body and interruption in the normal pattern of breathing. We often hear musicians complain that they tense their arms and joints much more when facing an audience than during their practising and they blame their 'nerves' for their failure to achieve a flawless performance. The reverse is also true: when the body is tense, nervous tension is also created (Grindea 1978).

Posture

Both the medical and musical professions agree that good posture plays a vital role. Disciplines such as Alexander technique, Feldenkreis, Tai-Chi, yoga and others are attracting more and

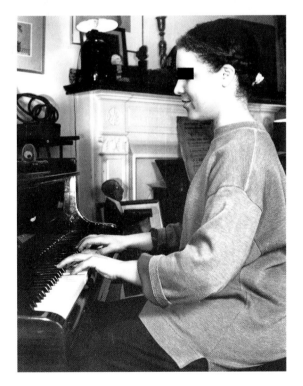

Figure 6

Posture: alignment of head, neck and back. See correct position of arms balanced away from the body (by courtesy of M de Gori).

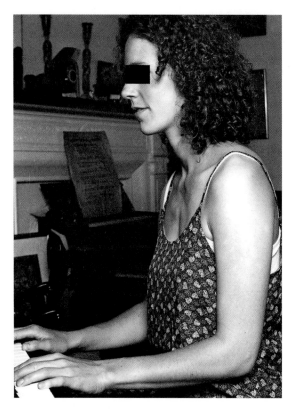

Figure 7

Incorrect position of shoulders forward, wrists inwards, arms too near the body, neck and head pushed forward (by courtesy of M de Gori).

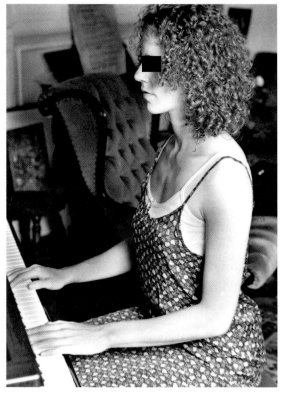

Figure 8

Shoulders (shoulder girdle) in correct position, sternum gently raised (relaxed) to correct the shoulder line – bringing head, neck and back in perfect alignment, arms suspended on each side of body, wrists in line with fifth fingers (by courtesy of M de Gori).

more followers and some are on the curricula of certain music colleges. All disciplines recommend a perfect alignment of head, neck and back, with an erect, vertical spine. This state of the body should be maintained throughout practising and in performance (Fig. 6).

Incorrect position of joints is another frequent occurrence which causes great pain in the wrists, elbows, shoulders, neck and back. The position of the shoulders and shoulder girdle is vital. Some players hold one shoulder higher than the other, or one or both brought forward several centimetres. Pain, 'pins and needles' or numbness in fingers is often the result. This is remedied through correcting the imbalances in posture, making sure that all

joints are in their correct position, each of which may need slight adjustments. The sternum should be raised gently. This immediately corrects any imbalance in the shoulders (Figs 7, 8).

Many pianists over-relax their arms, thinking that this is needed in good piano-playing. The arms hang down too low on each side of the body with a lot of weight in the elbows, which are then too near the body, creating a wrong alignment: the inner part of the forearm is in line with the thumb and this hinders the ease of movements along the keyboard. Arms should be held balanced, slightly away from the body, with elbows in line with the fifth finger, a position which facilitates all technical passages.

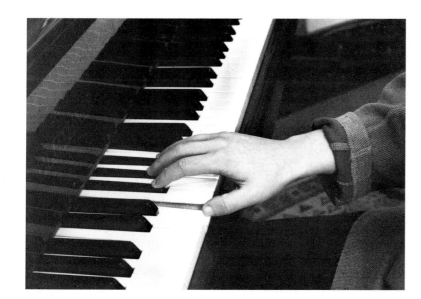

Figure 9

Correct position of hand with elongated fingers and wrist relaxed, in line with fifth fingers (by courtesy of M de Gori).

Thus the position of the wrist is one of the key conditions for a player to acquire skill in piano-playing (Fig. 9), as is the correct positioning of the thumb (Fig. 10) and fingers (Fig. 11).

Incorrect ergonomics – interaction between player and the instrument

Incorrect ergonomics is another source of physical problems. The player must feel at ease when playing the instrument, he must be 'attuned to it', and it must not be a struggle to achieve a good performance. Muscular co-ordination must be maintained throughout practising and in performance, and this demands highly specialized training. How is it possible to maintain freedom of muscular co-ordination when computer calculations show that the 22 muscles between the wrist and finger tips can produce no fewer than 2.4×10^{18} muscular combinations? While there is muscular contraction at the moment of tone production, this must not be carried beyond that moment. The answer lies in 'differential relaxation', when only the group of muscles needed for a certain movement should be active while the rest of the body remains alert, but in a balanced state (Lehrer 1985).

How can pianists' problems be treated and remedied?

Most problems seem to be caused by excessive negative tension. Since 'tension' is a physiological phenomenon which occurs in the mind and the body and is activated by the unconscious, it cannot be controlled by the conscious mind. Therefore, I approach this study by analysing not only the physical factors, posture, hands, fingers, knuckles, wrists, forearms, elbows, upper arms, shoulders, neck and back, but also the physiological processes involved, such as kinaesthesia, the state of balance of body and muscles, use of arm weight and muscular energy in piano-playing and freedom of breathing. I do not talk about 'relaxation'. A relaxed body cannot perform with ease and with freedom, just as an athlete cannot run in such a state.

Liberate the body and mind of any tension

Every musician who comes to the clinic has to learn, in the first instance, to liberate the body and muscles of any negative tension. We work in front of the mirror so that they observe their

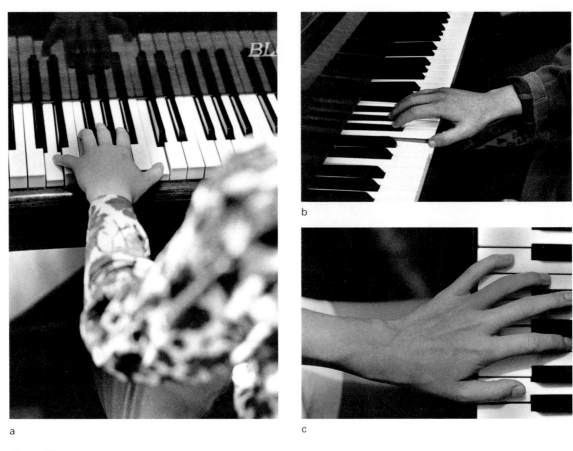

a   c

Figure 10

(a) Correct position of the thumb, resulting in a better position of wrist, elbow and shoulder; thus the arm moves with complete freedom in all directions. (b) Lateral view of correct thumb position. (c) Incorrect thumb position, which affects the position of wrist, elbow and shoulders (by courtesy of M de Gori).

posture and the line of shoulders and shoulder girdle, which is easily corrected by slightly raising the sternum. I introduce my own coping technique, 'Grindea technique',* which needs only a few minutes of concentration and which corrects any imbalance in the body through mental directives.

The player stands at ease, facing the mirror:

- Concentrate attention on the spine, ordering it to lengthen. This is not done through a movement, only through mental directives. One should experience the sensation of the head being gently lifted and placed towards the back, on the last vertebrae, bringing the head, neck and back into a perfect alignment.
- Exhale very slowly, whispering 'haaaaa' as long as possible; be aware of shoulders lowering, a state of relaxation in the diaphragm area, the arms getting longer and

*A video of the piano technique with explanatory brochure is available from the author.

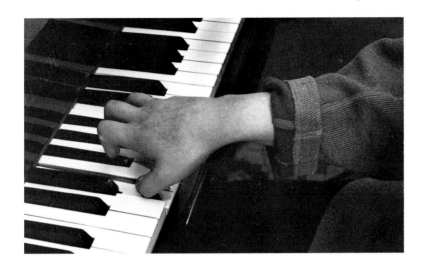

Figure 11

Incorrect position of wrist and fingers – this causes tendonitis and great pain when playing for various lengths of time (by courtesy of M de Gori).

heavier, with a great deal of arm weight flowing into the hands. Allow the body to take an in-breath. Be aware of the back expanding. Repeat this exercise two or three times.

• Concentrate attention on knees and ankles and imagine them very supple and flexible. One should experience the strange sensation of lightness as if the body is floating.

The player is experiencing an exhilarating feeling of well being. The 'Grindea technique' works on two levels: physically, by liberating the body of any tensions; and psychologically, by bringing stillness in the mind during those few minutes when practising the technique. Thus not only the body but also the mind is free of tensions.

To achieve this state of balance of the body and mind is easy and anyone can learn it in a few minutes. But to maintain it while practising and performing for hours is a very specialized study requiring slow practising with constant awareness of muscular freedom. This technique should be practised as often as possible so that it becomes an habitual state of body and mind.

Piano technique based on natural movements

Once the player has experienced the freedom from physical tension and has acquired a correct posture and is now also free of pain, he is ready to start working at the instrument.

He sits down comfortably, with erect back in line with the head and neck and with the right foot by the pedal. He places the hands, relaxed, on the keyboard with fingers elongated, in a natural position which are the natural movements in piano techniques (Fig. 7). If one observes the relaxed hands on the keys, one notices that the wrist is dropped. When the pianist moves his hands, relaxed, along the keyboard, the wrists are gently raised. Therefore, the message from the body is that the downward and upward movements of the wrist are the fundamental movements in piano-playing. Thus we work on a piano technique which uses these two movements. I believe it is essential that every keyboard player realizes when he is using a technique in harmony with the body and when this acts against the body, against the laws of nature.

The first and most important message from the body is that the wrists should never be locked, but should remain flexible through these two movements which get smaller and smaller, the faster one plays, while the arms remain in a state of balance. The pianist then learns to differentiate between when he has to use a great deal of arm weight for passages demanding a great volume of sound and when to use muscular energy, and between the need for a combination of these two physiological factors. This is, indeed, a specialized study, but any player can acquire it in one or two sessions. He soon realizes that the two fundamental movements are the only ones which release the tensions created while practising or performing. They help to achieve a balance between tension and relaxation.

Freedom of breathing

This is a vital physiological factor in instrumental playing. A good player breathes with the music, which flows through arms and hands into the keys and beyond. Pianists have a great capacity to stop breathing when approaching a passage which might give them worry and only exhale afterwards. Too late! I recommend playing with lips slightly parted; the pianist then has to breathe with the music. This is not only important but it is also very beneficial, as it is known that 'exhaling' counteracts the physiological reactions to anxiety. A long exhalation is nature's antidote to nervous and physical tensions.

The approach described above has helped countless musicians attending the clinic, but I do not believe that this is the only valid approach to piano-playing. Any school of piano technique can be used – and has been used successfully – if the muscular co-ordination is allowed to function freely. This explains perhaps why so many pianists, over the centuries, have been able to perform splendidly without developing physical problems, sometimes in spite of the teaching! The answer is that they play with all their muscles and joints in a harmonious state,

without any stiffness in the body. These are the players who, intuitively, use their body and arms in a 'natural' way.

References

Fischer S (1997) *Basics One*. London: Peters.

Grindea C, ed. (1978) Tensions in the performance of music – a symposium. Kahn & Averill, London; Pro Am Music Resources, New York.

Kember J (1995a) You and your guitar. Part 1. *Classical Guitar* **14**(3):24–5.

Kember J (1995b) You and your guitar. Part 2. *Classical Guitar* **14**(4):16–18.

Kember J (1995c) You and your guitar. Part 3. *Classical Guitar* **14**(5):16–18.

Kember J (1995d) You and your guitar. Part 4. *Classical Guitar* **14**(6):26–7.

Kember J (1995e) You and your guitar. Part 5. *Classical Guitar* **14**(7):31–2.

Kember J (1995f) You and your guitar. Part 6. *Classical Guitar* **14**(8):26–7.

Kember J (1995g) You and your guitar. Part 7. *Classical Guitar* **14**(12):26–7.

Lehrer S (1985) Beyond Ortman and Schultz. *ISSTIP Journal* **3**:26.

Markison RE (1990) Treatment of musical hands: redesign of the interface. *Hand* **6**:525–44.

Norris R (1993) *The musician's survival manual: guide to preventing and treating injuries in instrumentalists.* St Louis: MNP Music Inc.

4
Misuse and overuse

Christopher B Wynn Parry

We have asked well-known pedagogues to share their views of why musicians can suffer pain from poor technique and how it can be prevented. The reader is urged wherever possible to see first-hand with the help of a musical colleague how problems arise.

One of the most frequent clinical syndromes presenting in the musicians' clinic is the so-called upper limb pain syndrome. This used to be referred to as repetitive strain injury, but fortunately this term has now been dropped, for symptoms are not necessarily due to repetitive movements and there is no evidence of an injury or a strain. The patient typically complains of generalized aches and pains. These may be in the palms of the hands, in the depths of the thenar eminence, at the back of the hand or in the flexor or extensor surfaces of the wrist. They may later spread up to the muscles of the forearm and in severe cases even to the upper arms, neck, shoulder and thoracic and lumbar spine. Typically the symptoms are first felt after a prolonged period of practice, or after a very intensive spell of performing (Sakai 1992). The symptoms are usually felt in the hand and wrist. Later these symptoms can develop mid-way through a performance, and as the condition deteriorates, progressively sooner, until the moment the patient picks up the instrument, the symptoms develop. Eventually, all sorts of household activities become impossible and the patient is in almost constant pain. The outstanding feature of the condition is the marked discrepancy between the severe symptoms and the lack of physical signs. It is rare indeed to find any physical signs, other than some slight muscle tenderness. There is never any swelling of tendons, i.e. no true tendonitis, there are no colour changes, no crepitus and no limitation of movement or sensory loss, and true weakness is rare though there may be inhibition due to pain. No pathological findings have ever been reported and recently MRI scans have been conducted in typists who developed severe pain from typing and no abnormalities were found.

In our view, the condition is due to muscle fatigue and therefore has a biochemical basis. Biochemical changes are reversible, but if the condition becomes chronic, the patient will adopt various strategies to avoid pain and these may well lead to secondary disorders. The whole condition may become quite complex and requires very careful assessment whilst the musician is playing the instrument in order to unravel the particular strands of the problem. The condition is common also in students who are under stress and who are working against time and practising excessively and inefficiently. It can also develop when the musician is under stress, whether emotional, psychological or as a result of an unsatisfactory lifestyle, and as the fatigue increases and pain worsens, a vicious circle of pain, anxiety, tension, further muscular effort and more pain is established.

It is now well recognized that the chronic pain syndrome is a very real entity. Continuing nociceptic input to the spinal cord causes profound central changes with alterations of neuronal activity and neuronal networks, thus explaining why pain can be felt immediately the student resumes playing despite prolonged rest. There is a template of pain waiting to be alerted in the central nervous system. A very careful assessment must be made of any antecedent factors. The commonest causes are a marked increase in playing time, a more demanding repertory, a change of instrument, a change of teacher, the development of a new technique, and in the case of orchestral players a detrimental alteration in lifestyle. But perhaps the commonest cause is poor practice technique. It is very common for students to practise for many hours on end without a break for days or weeks on end. This leads to a chronic fatigue state and discomfort and pain in the particular muscles used.

John Williams, the famous guitarist (see Chapter 3), insists that no musician should practice for more than 20 minutes at a time. He should leave the instrument and carry out stretching exercises and general breathing exercises and in general put the muscles that have been tense on the stretch in the opposite direction in which they have been used.

A careful appraisal of the musician's lifestyle may also reveal a number of potent causes of local and general fatigue. The average orchestral musician, certainly in the United Kingdom, has a punishing schedule: most work three times as hard as their Continental counterparts for half the money and they have to supplement their earnings from the orchestra by session work and teaching. This often involves a great deal of travel, very long hours with rushed, inadequate meals and the inability to relax or take time off. In addition, there are frequently tensions within members of the orchestra and emotional and psychological problems are not uncommon. The stresses and strains that face orchestral musicians are discussed in detail elsewhere. Here it must be emphasized how important it is to listen carefully to the musicians' descriptions of their lifestyle and clues may well be found to the cause of symptoms. They can often be relieved by judicious advice about changing the pattern of their life or at least adopting strategies to cope with the tension and the stress. The help of an arts psychologist can be invaluable (see Chapter 16). It is wise to encourage the maintenance of as much physical and mental fitness as possible. In this respect, we are continually surprised at how little, if any, advice is given to music students in schools and even in the academies about the correct care of their bodies and the importance of getting fit for their instruments.

Playing an instrument is after all much like an athletic performance: one must become fit for the activity and this means having good joint flexibility, satisfactory muscle strength and stamina and the general fitness to cope with the various physical and mental strains of a life in music. Often tensions will arise due to overwork

or emotional stress and muscle tension results, causing musculoskeletal symptoms whilst both playing and practising.

It is important therefore that a musician has some form of physical discipline that can be brought into play under these circumstances, such that the body and the mind become relaxed. Many patients find the application of the Alexander technique (Rosenthal 1987) most helpful. We also favour simple yoga techniques or Tai Chi, and in special circumstances, particularly with dystonia, the Feldenkreis regime (Spire 1989). Whatever particular technique is adopted, the musician should appreciate the importance of his responsibility to keep himself as fit as possible and to practise whatever discipline he finds acceptable so that he can bring it into play in times of stress. This need be no more than simple relaxation techniques for 10 minutes or the application of some yoga technique or controlled breathing, but it is vital the musician feels he has a means of taking control over his body, rather than the body controlling him. If the physician senses that the patient's musculoskeletal symptoms are predominantly or even considerably caused by emotional or psychological stress, referral to an arts psychologist or counsellor can be most helpful. Such specialists are themselves musicians and understand the stresses and strains of a musician's life, and they can be invaluable in exposing the primary cause of tension and advising on relevant coping strategies. Many of our patients have totally lost all their musculoskeletal symptoms as a result of such skilful counselling and have returned to musical life with renewed enthusiasm.

The term overuse has been widely used to describe these upper limb pain syndromes. This to us implies that prolonged playing of a musical instrument might inevitably lead to problems. This is in fact not so. Lippmann (1991) has pointed out that there is no evidence that even intense and protracted playing in itself carries the risk of an overuse syndrome without a pre-existing injury or a chronic disease to disrupt normal play. He goes on to say that 'the majority of musicians who choose to spend their life with their instrument manage to emerge unscathed even after years of playing'. Our professional musical friends assure us that provided the technique is good, the mind calm and the lifestyle sensible, there is no need to suffer anything other than the odd aches and pains from a lifetime of music-making. Prevention, therefore, is the key to the management of this condition. A good sensible practice technique, attention to general health, regular holidays and diversified interests, in short the life of a happy and fit musician, should ensure that there are no problems.

There are some key periods in a musician's life when crises can arise; the first of these is when the student is preparing for exams for admission to music college and is likely to be practising very hard and getting into an emotionally tense state. There may also be problems with the parents. Some parents are excessively ambitious for their child and see in them the ability to achieve the ambitions which they were unable themselves to realize. The student thus becomes pressurized to succeed, works too hard with inadequate breaks and suffers pain. Alternatively, the parents may be hostile and resent the child having opportunities they did not have – the student again works excessively hard to try and impress. Also, it must be borne in mind that some students are unsure of their future and may be simply taking up music to please their parents and their tensions may find expression in musculoskeletal problems. An honourable way out of the impasse is the existence of arm pain or 'RSI'. Here the help of an arts psychologist or a sympathetic psychotherapist can be most helpful. Breakdowns are not uncommon in the first year at college when the student realizes that he is no longer the best in his school, but is competing with people with like or even better talents. It is here that bad practice techniques, excessive playing with inadequate rest and lack of attention to general health can cause musculoskeletal problems.

A student may well actually break down when preparing for final exams. We have seen patients who came to us with vague muscular aches and pains begging us for a certificate that they are unable to sit their exams because of RSI and asking for a postponement. Careful assessment of the degree to which symptoms are caused by emotional stress, poor technique, bad lifestyle or simply overpractice will usually settle the issue and allow reassurance that the patient has no underlying serious problem. Provided the various issues are addressed sensibly and calmly there is no reason why the patient should not take the exams. Clearly if there is profound psychological and emotional disturbance, then it would be wise to postpone the examination, but expert psychological guidance must be sought and the patient not treated with physical means as if it were a physical disability.

It is not uncommon for a well-established artist to have a crisis in mid-career. Each generation of keyboard and string players seems to be technically more brilliant than the last. There is a real fear among such artists, even of great international repute, that they will be ousted by the younger generation.

Many players feel that they must accept every engagement. If they do not do so, someone else will be ready to take their place. It is important to explain to musicians that they must guard their resources and look after their minds and bodies and it is pointless to undertake too many engagements which will produce general fatigue, a fall-off in performance and a vicious circle of muscular aches and pains and a serious impairment of their career. If a player has not previously had some form of physical and mental discipline to help him cope with such stresses, then we strongly recommend its adoption at this stage. Discussion with a wise guru whom they respect in their profession can often be most helpful.

In the acute stage of the upper limb pain disorder, rest may well have to be prescribed until the acute symptoms have subsided. Prolonged rest is counterproductive; skills are easily lost, confidence may be destroyed and patients who cannot practise their art easily become depressed. It may be necessary to prescribe anti-inflammatory or analgesic preparations for a few days, and appropriate aids to daily living to spare painful muscles and joints. But as soon as possible the musician should be encouraged to resume playing. This may be simply for 5 minutes at a time twice a day, gradually and slowly increasing the playing time. We advise them to keep a diary of the length of time they have been able to play and the onset of symptoms and how long those symptoms lasted. We exhort them to make friends with their instrument again and to play for sheer pleasure without any thought of preparing for exams or concerts. At the same time, the opportunity is taken to undergo a reassessment of technique, posture and general lifestyle, with particular attention to the musician's practice schedules and emotional state. At this stage, it may well be helpful to enlist the services of an arts psychologist or a counsellor if there is an underlying emotional problem, and those of a specialist musician experienced in the particular problems that their instrument can present with a view to overhauling their technique. We strongly deprecate the practice of advising musicians to rest for prolonged periods of time. We have heard of some clinics who have advised months or even years of rest, with advice to put the limb in a sling and not to use it for any activities. This attitude reveals an entire misunderstanding of the pathophysiology of the condition. Rehabilitation after a short period of initial rest is vital. We have seen patients in whom such prolonged rest has destroyed their career and has even led to disuse atrophy, stiff joints and, in extreme cases, reflex sympathetic dystrophy. Provided the condition is recognized for what it is and for what it is not, this multifaceted approach is almost always successful.

A review of the literature reveals that in the experience of long-standing specialist music clinics, well over three-quarters of patients with these performance-related problems are completely cured with appropriate treatment and advice on long-term performance practice. All emphasize that the sooner the musician is seen, the better, and all emphasize the importance of the multidisciplinary approach. Clearly, results will depend on the particular problem with which the patient presents. If there is indeed an orthopaedic problem, such as advanced arthritis, then continuing a music career may not be possible, but if it is clear that the symptoms are related primarily to poor technique, an inappropriate lifestyle or emotional tensions, provided these issues can be addressed satisfactorily, there is no reason why a musician should not resume a full career.

References

Lippmann HA (1991) A fresh look at the overuse syndrome in musical performance. *Med Probl Perform Artists* **6**:57–60.

Rosenthal E (1987) The Alexander technique. *Med Probl Perform Artists* **2**:53–7.

Sakai N (1992) Hand pain related to keyboard technique in pianists. *Med Probl Perform Artists* **7**:2.

Spire M (1989) The Feldenkreis method. An interview with Anat Baniel. *Med Probl Perform Artists* **4**:159–62.

5
Surgical evaluation: avoidance of pitfalls

Peter C Amadio

It is important to recognize that surgical evaluation of the musician's hand is in almost every way identical to the surgical evaluation of any hand. Any hand surgical evaluation must begin with an understanding of the patient and the role which the hand plays in that patient's career, activities of daily living, leisure activities and so forth. This is no more true for a musician than it would be for a homemaker, labourer or surgeon. The major difference is that the surgeon is likely to be familiar with most of the activities performed by the typical patient without explanation or demonstration. This may not be true for the musician, unless the surgeon has personal experience with the instrument upon which depends the musician's livelihood. Thus an introductory session for the purpose of understanding better the needs and requirements of the patient may be in order before making any specific surgical decision (Brandfonberner 1991; Graffman 1986). This session should include a review and if necessary observation of the method of play (Fig. 1) with a representative piece of repertoire; a history of lessons, practice schedules, performance schedules and any changes in technique, frequency or intensity of play.

Secondly of course one must confirm that a surgical condition actually exists from an anatomic or pathophysiological point of view. The patient may have been referred with the diagnosis of carpal tunnel syndrome; is that diagnosis correct? What evidence is there to support the diagnosis? Is it possible that multiple pathologies are present? If so which, if any, might be amenable to surgical treatment? Would a non-surgical approach be more appropriate and fit in better with the patient's needs?

In many cases patients are referred to a surgeon because other treatment modalities

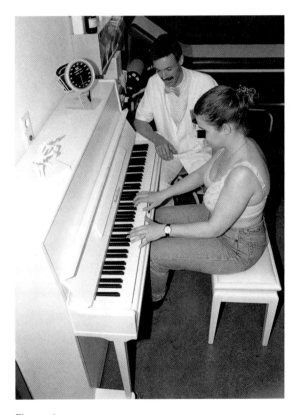

Figure 1

Ideal clinic facility for examination of musicians. Note the piano (by courtesy of Dr ABM Rietveld).

have not been of benefit and it is hoped that 'maybe surgery will help'. In my experience, this sort of referral represents an almost absolute contraindication to surgery. Not only is surgery

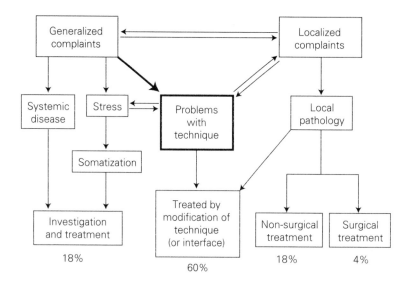

Figure 2

The complex interrelationships in musicians of generalized and localized symptoms and of generalized and localized pathology versus technical factors. Similar complex relationships exist between the need for adjustments of instrument or technique versus medical or surgical care. Of note is the small number who, on full analysis, require surgical care. These represent between 2 and 4% of all musicians presenting with upper extremity symptoms or injury. From Winspur and Wynn Parry (1997).

not likely to help; exploratory surgery and surgery for tentative indications have almost always, in my experience, proved to be a detriment. In musical performance, minute differences in finger position and in rates of fingering make all the difference between the virtuoso and the merely competent (Lockwood 1989). One of the main risks of surgery is that it might inadvertently distort the fine neuromuscular balance which creates these magical differences. In order to justify taking this risk, the surgeon and patient both need to have a fair degree of confidence that the current problem is already considerably worse than any difficulty which might be caused inadvertently by surgery, and further that non-surgical management is not likely to address the issue satisfactorily. These are difficult conditions to meet; one reason why, at least in my own clinic, surgical treatment of the musician's hand is infrequently chosen as an option (Amadio and Russotti 1990).

Perhaps the most common surgical indications will be in the area of acute trauma: because of the requirement for a high degree of hand function, anatomical reduction of fractures and anatomical repair of lacerated tendons and nerves will usually be in the patient's best interests. Techniques which permit early return to function, such as rigid internal fixation of

fractures, and early, specialized rehabilitation will often be beneficial. Other conditions which often require treatment are electrodiagnostically documented carpal tunnel syndrome and cubital tunnel syndrome, which do not respond to activity modification or other non-surgical therapy (Amadio and Russotti 1990; Caldron et al 1986; Crabb 1980; Winspur 1995).

As mentioned above, the surgeon's evaluation basically follows the medical evaluation of the musician's hand, but centres on determining whether a surgical condition is present. The first order of business is to determine what structure or structures have been injured or are dysfunctional. The second is to determine the aetiology of the problem. Is this traumatic, degenerative or neuromuscular? Is the focus central or peripheral? Only focally peripheral problems are likely to have a surgical solution (Fig. 2). Finally, what is the impact of the pathology on the patient's life and livelihood? If non-surgical treatments are possible, or if non-surgical adaptations can overcome the impediment, then usually these are to be preferred to any surgical treatment.

The evaluation is classic: a thorough history, followed by a general physical examination, and concluding with a detailed examination of the affected area. Specific areas of tenderness should be sought and there should be a general

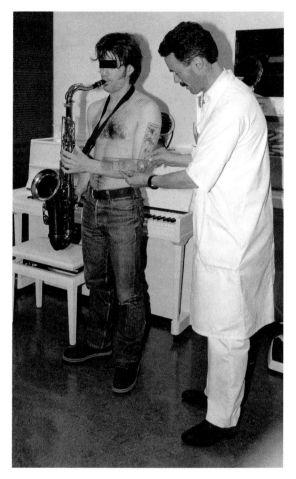

Figure 3

Examination of the musician patient: ideally this should be while they are undressed and playing (by courtesy of Dr ABM Rietveld).

and when or under what circumstances they occur, but also a general idea of what is wrong, whether the focus is likely to be central or peripheral, and whether it falls into a category where surgery is likely to be of benefit. At this point a more refined diagnosis can be obtained if necessary by further diagnostic tests. Routine X-rays may be helpful, as may be stress X-rays if joint instability is a concern. I have rarely found computed tomography, magnetic imaging or arthrography to be of particular benefit in the evaluation of the musician's hand, except in the setting of acute wrist injury. If a nerve compression syndrome is considered, then electrodiagnostic studies would be in order, both to assess the severity and to rule out any more proximal focus for any neuropathy. Particularly in a musician, proximal postures may well affect distal function, and what appears to be a carpal tunnel syndrome or ulnar neuropathy may in fact be found to be primarily a cervical radiculopathy or thoracic outlet syndrome, which would be amenable to postural modifications rather than surgical intervention (see Chapter 9).

There are many pitfalls along the way to trap the unwary. Most common is the tendency to equate localized pain or tenderness with a specific diagnosis. In the absence of swelling, erythema or pain on specific provocative tests, local pain or tenderness is more likely to represent undifferentiated myofascial pain than any more specific malady. Certainly the absence of erythema, heat and swelling should turn one away from any diagnosis of an inflammatory condition. Also common is the tendency to equate numbness or tingling with an entrapment of some nearby nerve. Neurological symptoms may arise from irritability anywhere along the course of a nerve. Awkward postures of the neck or shoulder are the source of many paraesthetic hands. All too many of these have been operated on. It is uncommon for a nerve compression disorder to require surgery in the absence of abnormal electrodiagnostic studies (see Chapter 9). Abnormal movements and cramps may be due to nerve compression disorders but are more often central, either habitual or dystonic; neither responds to surgery.

Finally, it cannot be overstated that the musician's social context must be taken into consideration. Anxiety, stress and depression are all known to magnify symptoms, often to the

evaluation of the ligaments for any laxity. This examination needs to be followed by an observation of the musician performing, if this is at all possible, followed immediately thereafter by repeat examination to see whether new areas of tenderness, instability or other impairment become evident (Fig. 3).

After completing a history and initial physical assessment, the surgeon should have a good idea not only where the symptoms are located, point where the surgeon can be deluded into believing in a falsely high level of anatomical severity. Addressing, or at least understanding, the underlying issues at home, school or work may go far in avoiding an unnecessary surgical procedure.

Once the history has been obtained and an examination and appropriate tests have been carried out, the surgeon should be able to provide a definitive recommendation whether a surgical solution is appropriate or not. If the decision is made to proceed with surgery, then techniques which hasten return to function should be favoured. Such methods include rigid fixation of fractures, high-strength suture of tendons, atraumatic decompression and arthroscopic management of intra-articular pathology. Just as important as the intra-operative surgical plan is the postoperative rehabilitation programme. This plan should be formulated in co-operation with a therapist skilled in the treatment of musicians, and should include an early return to at least limited work with the musician's chosen instrument. Ideally, the plan developed preoperatively will include an estimated schedule of return to both practice and performance.

If the decision is made to follow a non-surgical path, then a similar comprehensive rehabilitation plan will still need to be formulated; the sole difference is the absence of a surgical step.

It should be clear that both the art and science of medicine are called into action at a very high level when one evaluates and treats the injured hand of a skilled musician. A surgeon who is conscientious and understanding of the patient and the patient's needs, and is capable of assessing correctly the pathology, both anatomically and physiologically, is most likely to make the proper decision in advising for or against a surgical component of the overall treatment plan.

References

Amadio PC, Russotti GN (1990) Evaluation and treatment of hand and wrist disorders in musicians. *Hand Clin* **6**:405–16.

Brandfonberner A (1991) Special treatment for musicians? Some specific hazards of elective surgery. *Med Probl Perform Artists* **6**:37–8.

Caldron PH, Calabrese LH, Clough JD, et al (1986) A survey of musculoskeletal problems encountered in high-level musicians. *Med Probl Perform Artists* **1**:136–41.

Crabb DJM (1980) Hand injuries in professional musicians. *The Hand* **12**(2):200–2.

Graffman G (1986) Doctor, can you lend me an ear? *Med Probl Perform Artists* **1**:3–4.

Lockwood AH (1989) Medical problems of musicians. *N Engl J Med* **320**:221–4.

Winspur I (1995) The professional musician and the hand surgeon. In: Västamäki N, Vilkki S, Görasson H, et al, eds. *Proceedings of the 6th Congress of IFFSH*, Monduzi Editori: Helsinki, Bologna: 1207–11.

Winspur I, Wynn Parry C (1997) The musician's hand. *J Hand Surg [Br]* **22B**:433–40.

6
Surgical indications, planning and technique

Ian Winspur

Surgery on musicians' hands has traditionally enjoyed a poor reputation (Brockman et al 1990). This stems principally from Robert Schuman's unfortunate experiences attempting to obtain more power and flexibility in his ring finger by manipulations of the intertendinous connections of the extensor tendon to that digit. These ill-advised attempts may well have ended his career as a virtuoso pianist and condemned him to life forever in the shadow of his wife's pianistic talent. Whether his final complete mental breakdown can also be attributed to this would be pure speculation. Paderowsky, the great Polish pianist, also suffered a well-documented, very unfortunate experience at the hands of the surgeon for an inflamed hand (Zamoyski 1982). But in slightly more recent times, rumour also has it that Rubenstein suffered a lacerated flexor tendon while in the USA, which was repaired very satisfactorily using the modern surgical approach. However, he does not mention this episode at all in his lucid and candid biography, *My Many Years*, written shortly before his death in 1982. Also in recent times two short papers have been written, one on extensor tendon triggering and binding (Benetar 1994) and one on the mechanical problems of the extensor tendons when playing the E flat scale on the piano (McGregor and Glover 1988). Both of these papers show good results from surgical intervention using modern techniques and give grounds for guarded optimism for surgery on the musician's hand. Indeed, it is now conceded (Nolan 1993), although seldom in writing, by the few surgeons with experience on professional musicians' hands and their response to surgery that, given a clearly surgical problem and provided the surgery is performed with precision and skill and great attention is paid to each musician's very specific needs, a satisfactory result can be expected. We also now realize that musicians actually suffer many of the same common disorders as the general population of the same age and gender, and that some of these conditions require surgical solutions as they do in the general public (Winspur and Wynn Parry 1997). Our experience parallels that of other clinics in that between 4 and 6% of musicians presenting with recognized orthopaedic or rheumatological problems in an upper extremity will be candidates for surgery. The implications are, of course, much greater for musicians, for indeed their hands are their livelihood. Therefore the accuracy of diagnosis, analysis of need and disability and the precision in planning all need to be of the highest order to ensure a satisfactory outcome of surgery. Additionally, musicians do suffer an uncommon but unique condition for which surgery is absolutely contraindicated – focal dystonia (see Chapter 14). The treating surgeon must therefore be extremely vigilant, and indeed the assessment and care has of necessity to be attuned to the fact that it is a musician's hand which is being considered and the musician's career depends upon it.

Indications

'Indications' are formulations of benefit versus risk and form the basis of surgical decision making. When life and limb are at stake the formulations are clear and the indications firm. When considering operations for painful conditions, or some degree of loss of function, the formulations are muddied and indications much less concrete. When dealing with musicians with painful conditions, or in whom there is a slight loss of function – and a 1% fall off in performance may be sufficient to render the musician incapable of playing – the formulations are extremely difficult. Hence the most that can be said in general of surgical indications in musicians is that they are 'different' – in some cases looser, in others modified and yet in other conditions much stricter. There follow some examples for clarification.

Looser indications

• Trauma
• Post-traumatic reconstruction.

When dealing with injury to a musician's hand experience has shown that putting additional effort into achieving primary stable anatomical repair, even when relative contraindications exist, will be well rewarded by increased functional recovery. This also applies to the surgical handling of post-traumatic deformity, joint stiffness, tendon adherence and malunion. The same principles apply to secondary reconstruction of an established deformity. This theme is expanded and explained in Chapter 10.

Conditions requiring modified indications

• Benign tumours
• Dupuytren's contracture.

In musicians, small localized lesions, producing minimal local symptoms in a conventional sense, may lead to the development of extensive and sometimes widespread symptoms in the extremity or the whole upper body out of all proportion to the small basic lesion. An example of this is the small flexor sheath ganglions commonly seen in percussionists. These unbalance the drummer's technique, upset upper body co-ordination and positioning and very soon produce symptoms in the neck and shoulder. The drummer may not even suspect the basis of his difficulties. However, removal of the ganglion changes everything, the drummer

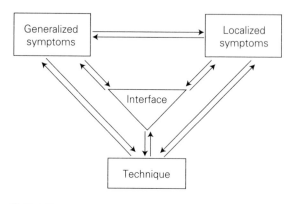

Figure 1

Relationship of symptoms, technique and the musical interface.

reverting to normal technique and posture (even with the suture still in place) and the distant symptoms settling rapidly. Conversely, generalized disorders, neck, back or shoulder pain, can unbalance the musician so that his technique changes to load excessively a localized unconditioned part where local symptoms occur. The treating doctor must be aware of this phenomenon and obviously the correct treatment in this situation must focus on the basic general cause. Yet a third confusing scenario may exist where minor imbalance or a maladjustment of the musical instrument may precipitate local loading and localized symptoms. In this situation surgery is absolutely contraindicated and an adjustment to the instrument needs to be made. These interrelationships are shown diagrammatically in Fig. 1.

Similar situations pertain in the case of small dorsal wrist ganglions which one would not normally consider treating. However, small wrist ganglions in musicians can cause symptoms and interfere or unbalance playing. When these small ganglions occur on the dorsum of a musician's wrist, it is worthwhile attempting to puncture them with a needle to aspirate fluid and to inject a steroid, even though the rate of recurrence is high. A small number will become asymptomatic or indeed disappear and the musician will be saved an operation. Persistent troublesome small dorsal wrist ganglions should be surgically excised in musicians if they are interfering with playing.

Metacarpal bosses are common in the general population and are seldom truly responsible for the symptoms claimed. The same is true of minor irregularities over the metacarpal heads (particularly the index) and apparent dislocating of extensor tendons within the extensor hood. However, we have seen two cases where painful dislocation of the extensor tendon to the index finger in the left hand of young viola players visibly occurred over a metacarpal boss while playing and the involved tendon was thickened and nodular. In both cases complete relief of symptoms (and dislocation) occurred with excision of the boss and contouring of the metacarpal base and adjacent dorsal carpus. This was performed when standard indications did not exist, but it was rewarded with the patients' rapid return to full-time asymptomatic playing.

Dupuytren's contracture, which predominantly affects males over 50 years of age, is naturally one of the commonest surgical problems seen in the musician population. Early contracting bands, particularly between the little and the ring fingers, cause significant difficulty to any musician playing an instrument on which wide span is required (piano or bassoon), even when digital flexion contracture does not exist. Even so, when causing functional difficulty to the musician, these early bands across the web space should be formally excised along with adjacent abnormal Dupuytren's fibrosis, even when conventional indications do not exist. Conversely, particularly in violinists, digital flexion contracture can exist with no functional loss even when joints are contracted to a degree where surgery is normally indicated. Under these circumstances in a musician, even if conventional indications exist for surgical release, no surgery should be performed until functional loss develops.

Conditions requiring stricter indications

- Nerve compression syndromes
- Tendonitis and trigger finger
- Tennis elbow.

The commonest site of nerve entrapment (see Chapter 9) both in the general public and among musicians is in the carpal tunnel at the wrist. When the median nerve is compressed at the wrist, a very typical set of symptoms and signs develop, but these can also be produced in a slightly modified form by prolonged positioning of the wrist in extreme flexion as is seen in many guitar players. They do not have carpal tunnel syndrome and they do not require surgery, but they do require re-education on their instrument to play in a more physiological position. A similar situation exists in the elbow, where the ulnar nerve passes around the fixed bony pulley, the medial epicondyle. Symptoms and signs of compression of the ulnar nerve can be produced in many patients by prolonged elbow flexion. In many cases modification of posture will solve the problem. However, a few musicians, forced to spend long periods with the elbow flexed, indeed show slowing of conduction on electrodiagnostic testing and surgical decompression of the ulnar nerve is sometimes indicated.

The symptoms of median nerve irritation or dysfunction are also seen in pianists following periods of intense playing when there is also evidence of tenosynovial swelling at the wrist and clinical signs of tenosynovitis in the fingers. In these circumstances, the median nerve is most frequently not directly compressed. Nerve conduction tests will usually be normal and the nerve does not require to be surgically released. Although nerve conduction testing has been shown to be slightly unreliable as a diagnostic tool for all patients with median nerve compression at the wrist, when dealing with musicians it is an essential screening test for true mechanical compression. Indeed the only method of clearly demonstrating nerve compression, so eliminating unnecessary and damaging surgical decompression in musicians, is by electrical testing of the nerve involved and clear demonstration of slowing of conduction in the segment of the nerve in question in comparison to other segments of the same nerve or the uninvolved contralateral nerve over the same segment. Hence one can state that when dealing with carpal tunnel syndrome or a possible ulnar nerve entrapment in a musician, strict indications should be applied and the nerve should not be surgically decompressed unless abnormal nerve conduction is demonstrated. The situation is less clear for radial nerve entrapment, however.

Tennis elbow is a chronic self-limiting painful condition of the common extensor origin which is surprisingly common among musicians. It seldom follows a specific sudden injury. When existing, the condition in musicians is constantly aggravated by the need to carry music cases, heavy suitcases, etc., particularly when on tour. Many cases will settle spontaneously if given sufficient time, with or without direct physical treatments such as massage or heat and with or without oral anti-inflammatory agents or indeed steroid injections into the lateral epicondylar area. In atypical cases other diagnoses should be excluded, particularly that of radial nerve entrapment. It is only after all non-surgical modalities have been exhausted and the condition allowed to settle over at least 12–18 months that this surgical approach should be contemplated. Following surgery, because of the mechanical nature of the surgical release and the physical requirements of playing virtually all musical instruments, recovery is slow and highly unpredictable.

Conditions with absolute contraindications to surgery

- Focal dystonia
- Exploratory surgery
- Conditions related to the musical interface.

Focal dystonia (see Chapter 14) represents a localized motor disorder manifesting in a single digit. It causes a painless spasm or inco-ordination of the digit which the musician will describe as a 'disobedient' finger. It is easily confused with localized triggering or intermittent extensor tendon binding. One must be very cautious. If dystonia is suspected, surgery is absolutely contraindicated as the additional insult only causes more scrambling and fragmentation of the patterns and programmes already disrupted in the midbrain.

There is no place for 'look and see' or exploratory operations for painful conditions in musicians. Similarly there is no place for exploratory operation for possible linkage between flexor tendons or extensor tendons unless under exceptional circumstances (see

Chapter 10). If local symptoms are related to an imbalance in technique or mechanical problems or to a change of instrument, a surgical solution is obviously contraindicated. Attention should be focused on the patient's technique and, if as in many cases is technically possible, adjustments made to the instrument.

Surgical planning

The surgical planning required when dealing with a musician's hand has to take into account both the pathology being dealt with and the very precise mechanical requirements and contact points for that musician and his instrument. This analysis must be completed before scalpel has touched skin. If the surgeon does not have detailed knowledge of the instrument involved, he can only plan accurately by examining the patient actually playing the instrument (Amadio and Russotti 1990). The musician cannot be expected to provide the accurate information required by description, and it is insufficient simply to question the musician and guess at the mechanical and anatomical details. The surgical planning however, should be focused in three areas:

- The siting of the incision to avoid critical tactile areas and to avoid sensory disruption to these areas
- The planning of the surgical exposure, operative technique and closure to facilitate very early return to limited playing
- The adjustment of any anticipated mechanical compromise to fit the playing position and the instrument rather than the conventional 'position of function'.

One would assume this type of planning and adjustment would be obvious, but that is not necessarily so, particularly if the musician is not examined with the instrument and, as sometimes required, accurate measurements taken.

The siting of incisions

The surgical approach and incision in a given situation is obviously dictated by the anatomical

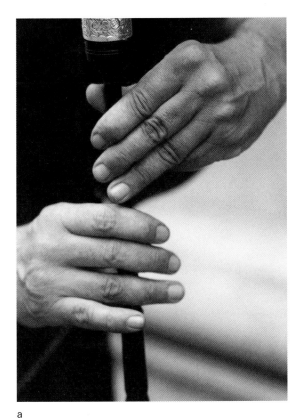 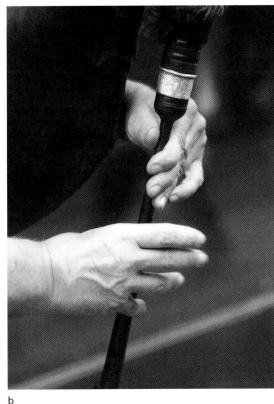

a   b

Figure 2

(a, b) The playing position of the bagpiper's fingers. Note the use of the middle segment of the finger, not the pulp, except for the right little finger.

requirements of the operation. It is also dictated by safety. But given these basic tenets, there is room for judgement. For instance, transverse incisions in the dorsal wrist creases give excellent access to the dorsal and radial aspects of the wrist including the radiocarpal joint itself and heal much more rapidly and with much less scarring than the longitudinal incisions crossing these creases. Similarly a mid-lateral approach to the proximal interphalangeal (PIP) joint heals much more rapidly and with much less morbidity than the more commonly used dorsal tendon splitting approach and in many circumstances will give better access to the joint. On the flexor aspect of the wrist and palm, longitudinal incisions crossing

the wrist crease directly will be very slow to heal and will remain thickened and hypertrophic for many months, restricting movement during this period. This is not a justification for approaching the carpal tunnel in musicians through small transverse incisions with poor visualization, or even approaching the carpal tunnel in these patients endoscopically with the slightly increased chance of serious nerve injury. But the surgeon should be encouraged, when possible, to avoid crossing the wrist crease (the standard short palmar incision for carpal tunnel release) or when crossing the wrist crease to do so with a step or zigzag in the incision to promote speedy healing and prevent scar hypertrophy. These nuances of

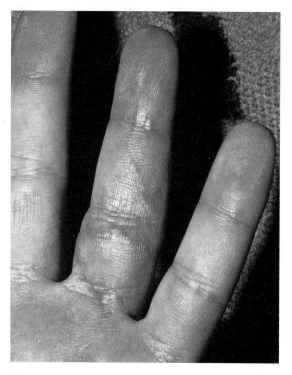

Figure 3

Tender scar from a classical Bruner incision over the critical middle segment in bagpipe players.

technique also apply to non-musician patients, but can truly make the difference when one is striving for an early return to playing.

When trying to avoid critical tactile areas, one has to examine the instrumentalist's technique and analyse digit by digit. Let us consider the Scottish (see Fig. 2) (or Irish or Greek) bagpipe player: the fingering on the chanter of these instruments is performed using the flexor aspect, middle segment of the index, long and ring fingers to provide a tighter air seal, and the pulp of the left thumb and the pulp of the right little finger. Hence the critical tactile areas which must not be violated are the flexor aspect of the three digits over the middle segments, the pulp of the left thumb and the pulp of the right little finger. When required surgically to approach structures on the flexor aspect of the digits, the standard modern approach is the Bruner zigzag incision or modification thereof (Fig. 3). This is incompatible with bagpipe playing when used on the index long or ring fingers and on these digits the incision, should this area need to be explored, has to be a non-standard, mid-lateral approach from the ulnar aspect elevating the neurovascular bundle with the flap and preserving all neurovascular connections, including fine sensory nerves to the middle segment of the flap (Fig. 4). However, the radial border and the pulp of the left thumb are

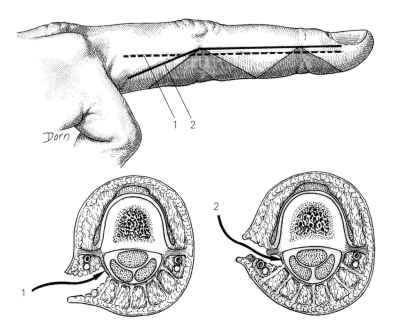

Figure 4

The mid-lateral approaches to the flexor aspect of the digit: either parallel to the midlateral line (1) or in a zigzag fashion (2). Approach 2 – elevating the flap and neurovascular bundle – is the only functional approach in bagpipe players. From Tubiana et al (1990).

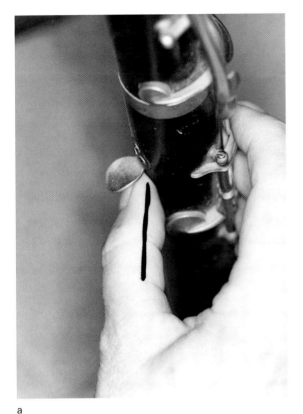
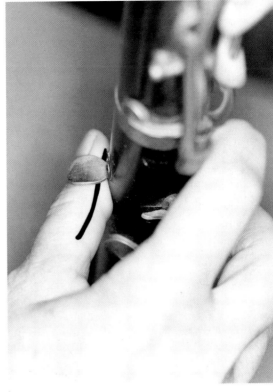

a   b

Figure 5

(a,b) The right thumb of a clarinet player. The marking indicates a poorly planned incision for exploration of the thumb pulp or the IP joint.

also used to finger the instrument and therefore this area is critically important and should not be violated. Additionally the pulp of the right little finger is critical in the playing of the Scottish bagpipe. Dupuytren's contracture, for hereditary reasons, affects Scottish pipers and is known as the 'curse of the MacCrimmons'. It does affect the little finger with unfortunate frequency and makes playing impossible. Fortunately the standard volar 'Z'-plasty approach on the little finger does not violate the critical tactile areas on that digit (the middle segment is not critical) and it can therefore be used and should allow clear visualization and dissection of the digital nerves and the deforming Dupuytren's tissue.

There are other examples of critical areas:

- The tips of the pulp of the digits on the left hand in string players
- The ulnar border of the right thumb in clarinet and oboe players (Fig. 5)
- The pulp of the thumb, index, long and little fingers in the right hand or bowing hand of string players
- The radial and ulnar borders of the ring and long fingers in drummers.

Each individual musician might also have their own non-standard modification of technique which might highlight a specific area.

Early return to playing

For a musician, playing is an essential life function and to be denied that or to be physically incapable has profound implications. They feel they have completely lost their raison d'être. Absence from playing has never been shown to be therapeutic and certainly not in the postoperative period. For professional musicians, whose livelihood depends on their ability to play, it is indeed therapeutic for them to be able to demonstrate to themselves at a very early point postoperatively that they still can play, that they have not lost their skill and that their fine programming and 'memory' which they have acquired through years of practice has not deserted their injured fingers. In this regard, it is important that the surgeons do all possible to facilitate an early return to limited playing. In certain circumstances, for example following flexor tendon lacerations and repair in zone 2, the poor tensile strength of the early repair and the biological and mechanical limitations of tendon healing will prevent return before the 8- to 10-week point. But in other situations attention to the location and direction of incision and accurate tension-free wound closure should allow early return to limited playing as early as 3–4 days. Indeed in our experience, the return to limited playing (5 minutes 3–4 times per day) on the fourth or fifth day postoperatively seems to be ideal (see Table 1).

When releasing Dupuytren's contracture the closed methods facilitate earlier return to playing than do the open palm techniques and therefore should be favoured in musicians. Similarly, skin grafts are used in secondary Dupuytren's releases in conjunction with healthy tension-free 'Z'-plasty flaps of non-involved skin to allow rapid wound healing and early return to playing. Again, in a small series of professional musicians undergoing Dupuytren's release (both primary and secondary), the average time absent from playing was 2 weeks (prolonged slightly by the grafted recurrent cases), although the primary releases usually return to limited playing at 5–7 days. All returned to full performance in an average time of 6 weeks. In cases of unstable fractures, open reduction should be considered earlier than with non-musicians. The fixation technique should be stable (Fig. 6) and allow early motion, and ideally k-wires and Steinman pins should not be left protruding through the skin, causing irritation and limiting motion. K-wires also should not be driven through or left protruding to form tender scars on critical tactile areas, particularly the very tips of the fingers on the left hand in string players. If motion needs to be limited or protected, this should be achieved by light custom-made thermoplastic splints positioned and shaped to allow playing of the instrument wherever possible.

However, one must be cautious and guard against too excessive or enthusiastic early playing or premature return to full rehearsal or performance. If the patient is not truly fit, and this means fully mobile and pain free, if full performance is attempted too early the musician will quickly develop compensatory mannerisms and alterations in technique. These may work well in the short term, but if they become permanently imprinted they will eventually be manifested in symptoms elsewhere due to overall misuse of the musician's limb. Early limited simple playing is therapeutic, premature performance can be permanently damaging.

Table 1 Duration of postoperative recovery necessary in 34 professional musicians (32 returned to full-time playing, 1 was lost to follow-up, 1 was unable to play). Follow-up: 3 months to 12 years

Medical condition	No.	Weeks off instrument	Weeks to full performance
Trauma	7	5.4	8.4
Dupuytren's	8	2.4	5.3
Tumours	8	0.8	3
Carpal tunnel syndrome	4	1.8	6
Arthrodesis	3	3	13
Cubital tunnel syndrome	2	6	12
By instrument			
Piano*	11	4	7.4
String*	10	2.5	7.5
Guitar	4	2	4.5
Other	7	2.5	5

*Prolonged by trauma, cubital tunnel syndrome and arthrodesis cases

Anatomical compromise

The aim of modern surgery is to achieve repair or cure without residual anatomical compromise.

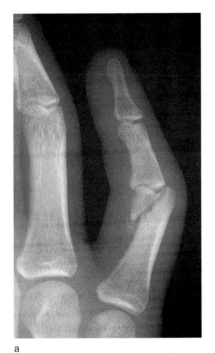

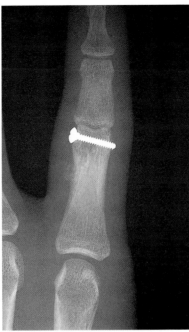

a   b

Figure 6

(a, b) Stable compression screw fixation of a displaced shortened rotated phalangeal fracture allowing very early mobilization (by courtesy of Dr G Crawford).

However, even in the best circles, certain injuries or certain operations will be followed by predictable loss of movement. Certain pathological conditions can only be treated surgically by deliberately reducing or eliminating the motion in a joint by tenodesis or arthrodesis – this is not necessarily a career-ending step for a professional musician, although it may prevent playing at the highest levels. In these situations, where loss of motion is to be expected, every effort should be made to ensure that the compromised joint, digit or limb is positioned in the functional playing position for that musician. If we consider the distal interphalangeal (DIP) joint of the digits in pianists, the great variation in playing positions can be highlighted. The 'standard' playing position is with the fingers slightly flexed and the DIP joints flexed at 30°–40°. However, whenever one observes professional pianists, both jazz and classical, one sees that the position of the fingertip and the DIP joints changes while playing, depending on the position of the hand and the type of sound being produced at that moment. The positioning is also dependent on the size of the musician's hand, the length of the fingers and the style of playing. Indeed the position can vary from hyperextension (Jelly Roll Morton) to tight flexion (Count Basie). There is no true standard position. Therefore, in considering the potentially compromised distal joint in a given pianist, the required average playing position of that particular joint can only be identified and measured while playing. If surgery is planned and loss of motion anticipated as a result, planning must be done at the piano, even if this requires a visit to the local piano showroom or the patient's home or practice studio.

In the string instruments the variations are less extreme, although the actual position of the distal joint when playing is maybe more extreme, particularly on the viola. In woodwind instruments the positions are again less extreme, but full span with hyperextension may be required for the right little finger on the bassoon and some woodwind players actually finger in a

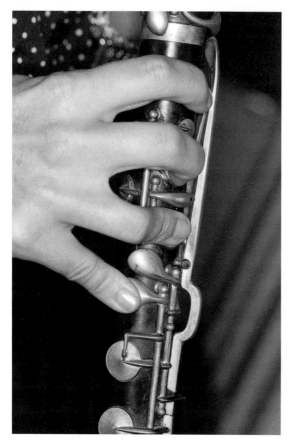

Figure 7

Common positioning of the right ring and little fingers in woodwind players. Note the 'physiological boutonnière' position of the ring finger pip joint.

mild boutonnière position for the right long and ring fingers.

When surgically arthrodesing or tenodesing a joint (Chapter 7) exact measurements have to be taken on the musical instrument and reproduced accurately at the time of surgery. For example, a patient, a violinist with compromised flexion of the DIP joint of his left index finger, required 50° of flexion to finger the E string measured preoperatively. This was accurately reproduced in surgery and satisfactory playing achieved.

When residual loss of motion is anticipated from a periarticular injury or adjacent tendon injury, one can try and adjust the anticipated slight loss to accommodate a particular need. For example, in considering the closed treatment of a closed secondary boutonnière deformity in the left ring finger of a viola player, two primary functional requirements can be identified from knowledge and observation of viola playing – 95° of PIP flexion and 60° of DIP flexion are necessary but full extension of the PIP joint is not.

The boutonnière deformity, even if mild and with a passively mobile PIP joint, is not compatible with the DIP flexion requirement and has to be corrected (Zancolli 1979). This requires 4–6 weeks of extension splinting of the PIP joint with the DIP joint free and maximally and continuously actively flexed. The next stage of treatment requires rapidly regaining PIP flexion and maintaining DIP flexion, but at the possible expense of 10–15° of PIP extension provided the boutonnière deformity does not show signs of recurring. Indeed, in the case being discussed, the functional requirement was achieved 12 weeks after starting initial splinting but with a final 15° loss of full extension of the PIP joint which was completely compatible with playing. Similarly, in the treatment of mallet deformity, if full flexion is mandatory for playing, this can be achieved at the risk of slight loss of extension. The reverse, where required can be achieved by excessively prolonged extension splinting at the expense of full flexion.

In the surgical management of Dupuytren's contracture, when full extension is not required for playing, the surgical emphasis should be on obtaining functional release, prevention of early recurrence by complete but safe clearance of contracting bands, protection of critical digital nerves and digital vessels and securing primary wound healing. The emphasis should not be on obtaining absolute complete full extension at risk to any of the above, nor at risk to functional flexion, nor indeed at risk to the tip of the digit itself from vascular compromise.

Surgical procedure

Anaesthesia

Musicians, as a group, are distrustful of doctors and surgeons. They only present with reluctance and, while not afraid in the classical sense, they are highly sceptical and resent any loss of control. For this reason, they generally much prefer local to general anaesthetic and where circumstances allow, which is certainly for most non-emergency hand surgical operations, surgery on a musician's hand should be performed under local anaesthesia. There are two other important advantages to performing hand surgery under local anaesthesia. First, rehabilitation begins the moment the operation has ended. This is because the patient is clear minded, feels he or she has participated in the experience and is anxious to proceed and to follow any next step accurately. The next step is, of course, to realize that they are not unwell or damaged and that they must continue with their full lives, even though for a few days they cannot use their hand or play and must elevate the hand conscientiously.

The second advantage is of course just this. From the moment the operation ends, particularly if not using brachial plexus blocks, the patient can maintain absolute high elevation of the hand (held resting on their heads 40 cm higher than the heart). It is this very early high elevation, which in our experience, and in the experience of others, substantially reduces the postoperative swelling and pain in patients operated on under local anaesthesia, as opposed to those undergoing general anaesthesia, even those maintained in a hospital bed with the hand elevated in a roller towel for the first 24 hours and then in a sling.

The specific techniques of local and regional anaesthesia are outside the scope of this book. Our particular preference for most non-emergency hand surgical operations, however, is a modified Bier block (see Appendix I). This has given very reliable, safe, complication-free anaesthesia in over 5000 cases personally and in well over three times that number for surgical colleagues with whom I have worked closely over the last 17 years.

Modification of surgical technique

Standard atraumatic surgical technique, as used in all hand surgical operations, is similarly used on musician's hands. Primary wound healing with the minimum of postoperative swelling is essential to achieve the early functional return

which is necessary in these patients. Specific alterations in surgical technique are only applicable in three areas:

- Siting and direction of incisions
- Protection of vulnerable sensory nerves
- Anatomical repair in distal nerve injury.

Atraumatic technique with very delicate tissue handling minimizes tissue damage, which delays healing and forms excessive scar. The use of appropriate magnification reduces the chances of inadvertent injury to undamaged structures and minor sensory nerves and increases the accuracy of repair. It also facilitates repair of the much smaller, more distal tissues and structures, particularly digital nerves and their branches. Because of the dramatic benefits from endoscopic surgery in operations where the surgical approach causes so much additional injury itself (knee, shoulder, gallbladder), there is a great temptation to perform other less suitable operations through keyholes. Musicians associate surgery and scars with morbidity and will anxiously inquire about the availability of endoscopic and 'laser surgery'. However, the surgical approaches to the hand and wrist do not cause the morbidity associated with these three previously mentioned areas and therefore there is little to be gained by the endoscopic approach. Indeed, the endoscopic techniques used for the release of the carpal tunnel are known to have a slightly higher incidence of nerve injury – a career-ending event for a musician – even in experienced hands. For this reason alone, the simple straightforward open approach through a short palmar incision, not crossing the wrist crease, is probably the most appropriate option when releasing the carpal tunnel of a musician, and when this is properly explained, the musician will freely accept this recommendation. There are other reports of the use of the endoscope for decompressing the ulnar nerve at the elbow, and indeed when dealing with a musician similar provisos again pertain. Wrist arthroscopy, however, in certain specific situations has been shown to be of both diagnostic and therapeutic value and is indicated in musicians in certain very specific circumstances. These would include the accurate reduction of intra-articular wrist fractures and also the diagnosis and repair in some circumstances of intercarpal dissociations. Elbow arthroscopy is of particular value and minimizes the morbidity in the handling of intra-articular pathology, particularly the removal of loose bodies which may be causing troublesome locking and pain or recurrent synovitis related to chondral lesions of the radial head or capitelum.

In the management of fractures, when the fracture is unstable or intra-articular and displaced, in the musician there is every reason to seek stable anatomical reduction. Again the basic techniques of fracture fixation are used and ideally internal rather than external fixation should be utilized, to allow very early range of motion and the ability to return to early playing of the instrument.

Intra-articular fractures of the small joints of the hand where displaced should ideally be treated by compression screw fixation and early mobilization and nowhere is this seen more than in the Bennett's fracture in a musician. Indeed, there is not a modern musical instrument (with the exception of the trumpet and the related coronet and flugel horn) in which both thumbs are not used. Therefore early anatomical reduction of the Bennett's fracture using the single compression screw should be the treatment of choice for this fracture in musicians. Displaced phalangeal and metacarpal fractures with even the slightest suggestion of shortening and rotation and digital overlap should again be treated by open reduction and ideally by compression screw fixation, if appropriate (Fig. 6). If k-wires or Steinman pins are required, these should be cut short so as not to interfere with early mobilization.

In summary, when dealing with the musician's hand or arm for a surgical condition, surgical indications are different, surgical planning must be detailed and accurate and surgical technique precise. The results, provided indeed a localized surgically remediable condition is the source of the trouble, can be expected to be as good as, if not better than, the results seen for similar conditions treated surgically in the general population.

References

Amadio P, Russotti GM (1990) Evaluation and treatment of hand and wrist disorders in musicians. *Hand Clin* **6**:405–16.

Benetar N (1994) Radial subluxation of the connexus intertendineus at the little finger in musicians. *J Hand Surg* **19b**:81–7.

Brockman R, Chamagne P, Tubiana R (1990) The upper extremity in musicians. In: Tubiana R, ed. *The Hand*, vol. 4. WB Saunders: Philadelphia: 873–85.

McGregor IA, Glover L (1988) The E flat hand. *J Hand Surg* **13a**:692–3.

Nolan W (1993) Surgical treatment of acquired hand problem. In: Bejjani F, ed. *Current Research in Arts Medicine*. Cappella Books: Chicago: 319–22.

Tubiana R, McCullough CJ, Masquelet AC (1990) *An Atlas of Surgical Exposures of the Upper Extremity*. Martin Dunitz: London.

Winspur I, Wynn Parry CB (1997) The musician's hand. *J Hand Surg* **22B**:433–40.

Zamoyski A, *Paderewski* (1982) Athenium: New York: 74–5.

Zancolli EA (1979) Pathology of the extensor apparatus of the fingers. In: Zancolli EA, ed. *The Structural and Dynamic Basis of Hand Surgery*. JB Lippincott: Philadelphia: 79–103.

7
Specific conditions

Cervical spondylosis

Christopher B Wynn Parry

In the older musician, cervical spondylosis may present with pain in the shoulder and the forearm and can be wrongly diagnosed as a technical problem. As well as the standard physiotherapy techniques for relieving pain, the musician must be given detailed advice on neck discipline – choice of pillows at night, avoidance of holding telephone between neck and shoulder, the means of avoiding stress on touring and long coach journeys and the importance of relieving stress on the neck by the judicious use of straps, harnesses, shoulder rests, etc (Fig. 1). It is wise when appropriate to ensure that vision is satisfactory, with correct spectacles being used. If not, advice from an oculist should be obtained as peering forward to read the score can cause chronic neck pain.

Thoracic outlet syndrome (TOS)

Christopher B Wynn Parry

A not uncommon presenting symptom among musicians is pain spreading down the inner aspect of the arm with paraesthesias in the ring and little finger and clumsiness and difficulty in playing their instrument. The arm may feel heavy and after prolonged playing the musician complains that he does not know what to do with his arm. Lifting and carrying causes pain. Abduction of the arm, particularly playing on the G-string on the violin, can cause pain.

The classic cervical rib syndrome, with wasting of the intrinsic muscles in the hand and sensory loss, is rare, but in most of the large series of upper limb problems in musicians reported, some 9–13% of patients present with the symptoms of compression of the roots of the brachial plexus at the thoracic outlet without overt neurological signs. It is commoner in tall, thin people with long sloping shoulders and is frequently associated with heavy instruments which put a traction strain on the plexus.

The majority of tests described as specific for this condition (see Chapter 9) are unhelpful, but Norris (Norris 1993) finds the 'elevated arm test' helpful in some patients. He asks the musicians to hold the arms overhead with shoulders and elbows bent at 90°. He then asks the musician to open and close the hands for 60 seconds. If there is pressure on the plexus, pain should be reproduced. Electrical tests will help in excluding local entrapment neuropathies, such as median nerve irritation at the wrist or ulnar nerve lesions at the elbow, but the diagnosis is primarily clinical. If a cervical rib is demonstrated on X-ray, this is helpful, but most patients have normal X-ray findings. We find the most useful sign is reproduction of symptoms by pressure over the root of the plexus on one side and not the other. Modern high-resolution MRI of the root of the neck or MRI angiography of the thoracic outlets is so accurate that a static cause can virtually be excluded.

Most patients will respond to a course of shoulder-raising exercises to build up the power of the shoulder elevators. Careful instruction in avoidance of stress with the judicious use of straps, harnesses, etc. and a general fitness programme is recommended. If symptoms do not subside with these simple measures, then referral to a specialist unit for sophisticated studies is indicated. Lederman (1987) reported on 17 patients with classic signs and symptoms of TOS. All but two responded dramatically to

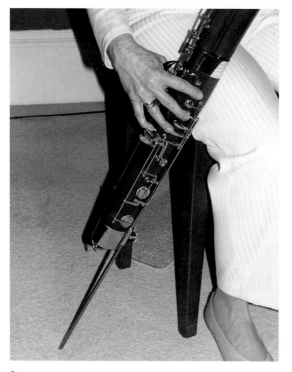

a

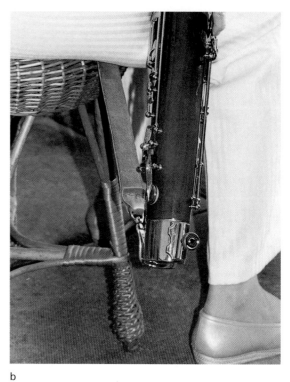

b

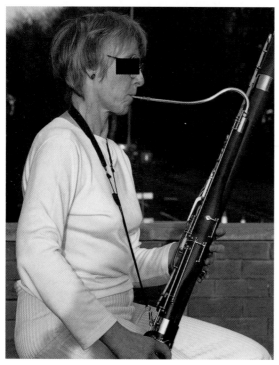

c

Figure 1

(a) Bassoon spike and (b) chair strap to eliminate neck straps (c) for those with cervical spondylosis (by courtesy of Dr J Riley).

conservative therapy. The Alexander technique is particularly helpful in these patients. Only two required surgery.

Rheumatoid arthritis

Christopher B Wynn Parry

Bird and Graham (1991) reported that fewer than 5% of patients referred to a musician's clinic will have one of the many sorts of arthritis. They point out that this is not necessarily career-threatening. With careful management of the rheumatic disease, it is surprising how many patients with quite severe generalized osteoarthritis or rheumatoid arthritis affecting the hands are able to continue playing. They point out that the relatively slow progress of these diseases allows the musician plenty of time to acquire minor changes of technique that may be required. Wynn Parry and Stanley (Wynn Parry and Stanley 1993) pointed out how early synovectomy of flexor tendons and the small joints of the hand can result in spectacular relief of symptoms and return of function. It is certainly worth bearing this point in mind and referring a musician whose swollen tendons and joints are not responding to the standard medical treatment to a skilled hand surgeon who understands musicians' problems. In the chronic stage, it may be necessary for the musician to modify his repertory and perhaps use a non-steroidal anti-inflammatory preparation, either locally or by mouth, before a demanding performance. It is particularly important that the musician with arthritis warms up well before starting practice or performance. General assessment is vital and the correction of any anaemia is a priority.

Osteoarthritis

Ian Winspur

Osteoarthritis presents most frequently in middle age as pain in the base of the thumb from carpometacarpal (CMC) arthritis. This of course seriously affects both string players and keyboard players, but a great deal can be done particularly in the early stages to minimize symptoms. We advise the patient to apply slow sustained traction to the thumb with the other hand several times a day. This stretches the capsule and often relieves pain for many hours, allowing practice and performance. At a later stage a judicious steroid injection can give many months of freedom from pain. There are a variety of surgical procedures now available to reduce symptoms. Again, referral to a hand surgeon who understands musicians' problems is vital.

Although an X-ray survey of musicians' hands demonstrated an unusual pattern of cysts in the distal finger joints, no clear correlation has ever been established between long-term playing of a musical instrument and the development of degenerative arthritis in the joints of the hands (Lambert 1992). Yet osteoarthritis of the hands, either as part of a patient's predisposition to develop generalized degenerative osteoarthritis with aging, or secondary to old trauma in a specific joint, is common enough in the general population for one eventually to be faced with a musician suffering from painful, stiff or unstable joints in the hand or finger from osteoarthritis.

The diagnosis is made by clinical examination – a painful, stiff, swollen or unstable joint, with provocation reproducing symptoms – and is confirmed by X-ray. As part of the pathological process, synovial inflammation (synovitis) may be present, and is indicated by boggy swelling and redness around the joint. On the dorsum of the dorsal interphalangeal (DIP) joints, enlarged tender nodules of granulation tissue and synovitis surrounding small osteophytes may be present (Heberden's nodes).

Assessment of the musician, however, is not complete until one has checked for more proximal areas of involvement, particularly of the neck and shoulder, for indeed subtle loss of motion or stiffness in these areas may have profound effects distally in relationship to their playing. One has also to analyse the particular joint involved in relationship to the patient's instrument and playing techniques. One may find that one painful joint is not functionally involved, but only a distraction, whereas another involved joint is in fact critical. Also modification of the interface is frequently of prime importance when dealing with isolated osteoarthritis of finger joints (see Chapter 3).

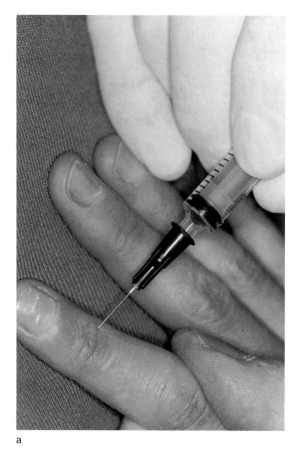

a

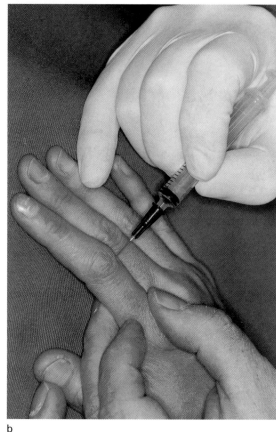

b

Figure 2

Approach and technique for injecting DIP (a) and PIP (b) finger joints.

Clinical details

The commonest joints to be involved in the osteoarthritic process are the distal joints of the fingers, the carpometacarpal (CMC) joints of the thumb and some of the intercarpal joints. The treatment required depends on:

• Amount of synovitis present
• Degree of articular degeneration (X-ray changes)
• The specific functional requirements of that joint in that musician.

Synovitis

If a joint is clearly the site of active synovitis and is painful, the condition can frequently be controlled, either by oral non-steroidal anti-inflammatory agents (NSAIDs) or more specifically and most frequently overlooked, by direct steroid injections into the joints (Palmieri et al 1987). A single injection into a phalangeal joint or CMC joint can give many months of complete relief and, although it does not substantially alter the course of the disease, if the synovitis can be controlled, the joints can be rendered painless

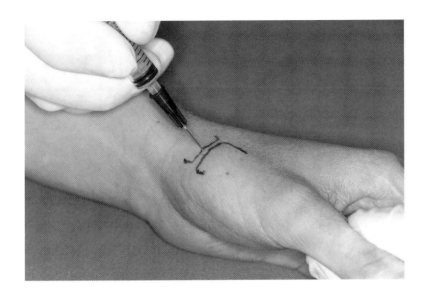

Figure 3

Technique for injecting the CMC joint. Note longitudinal traction maintained on the thumb by the operator's non-injecting hand to open up the joint space and allow easier entry into the joint.

and mobile even in the face of substantial X-ray changes. Nowhere is this more commonly seen than in the CMC joint.

Injection technique

When injecting the interphalangeal (IP) or CMC joints fine needles should be used and the joints should be approached from the dorsolateral or dorsomedial aspects (see Figs 2 and 3). Approximately 0.5 ml of a mixture of 0.5% bupivacaine hydrochloride and methylprednisolone (40 mg/ml) mixed in equal proportions is injected into the dorsal sulcus deep to the extensor mechanism. When the CMC joint is being injected a small short 26 gauge needle is used after the joint space has been identified dorsally by palpation and the interval between the metacarpal base and the trapezium has been widened by longitudinal traction on the thumb (Fig. 3). One millilitre of the mixture is injected into this joint.

Heberden's nodes

Heberden's nodes can at times become acutely painful and distracting. The underlying process of synovitis and inflammation will eventually burn itself out, but this takes many months. When active painful inflammation involves a critical digit on a musician, it may not be possible or acceptable to await the slow, natural resolution of the process. In these circumstances, steroid injection into the node may produce relief and, failing this, surgical excision, provided it is performed with skill respecting the very thin skin in the area and the close proximity of the nail-fold and the germinal matrix of the nail-bed, will provide near instant relief which should be permanent.

Articular degeneration

Patients are seen with severe degeneration apparent on incidental X-ray but with very little in the way of symptoms and functional loss, and vice versa. When pain, loss of mobility or instability are present in the face of deterioration on X-ray, one is faced with a very difficult problem in a musician. If synovitis is present and pain is a predominant symptom, intra-articular steroid injection may provide marvellous respite. When synovitis is not present, one is then faced with a number of options:

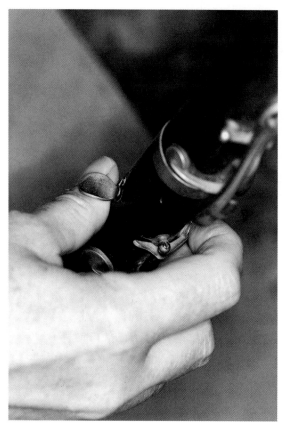

Figure 4

Weight of clarinet being taken on IP joints of the right thumb.

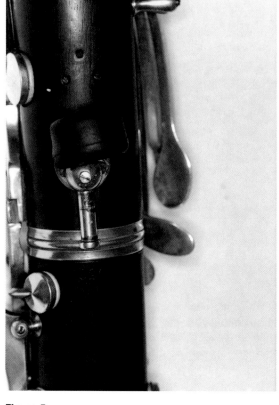

Figure 5

Modified thumb post spreading the load on to the proximal phalanx.

- Protective splint
- Modified instrument
- Arthrodesis
- Arthroplasty.

In the case of CMC arthritis (Nolan and Eaton 1989), when the thumb provides an important but static supporting role in woodwind players, a small custom-made thumb spica splint may be all that is required (see Chapter 11). When this joint is involved in a more active role, for example the right bowing thumb on a cellist, a change from a French to a German bow may solve the problem. In the case of IP arthritis in the right thumb of woodwind players (or traumatic synovitis) (Fig. 4), modification of the thumb post spreading the load on to the proximal phalanx may provide a solution (Fig. 5). If a distal finger joint is slightly unstable, or has a slight flexion or angular deformity, minor repositioning of the keys on woodwind instruments may be effective.

When the joint is functionally important and is painful and unstable one is left with the options of surgical arthrodesis or arthroplasty. Neither of these operations need necessarily be career-ending, although it is doubtful whether one could remain at full concert soloist level following one of these operations. When planning arthrodesis of one of the IP joints, it is important that the musician's playing position be

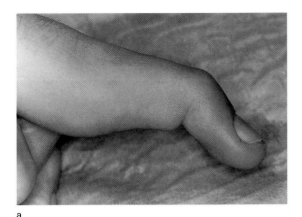
a

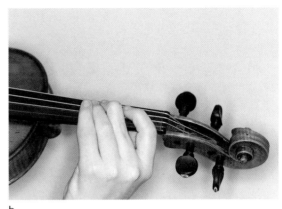
b

Figures 6–13

Localized monoarticular arthropathy of PIP joint of left long finger with fixed swan-neck deformity and abnormal finger-ing. Preoperative use of malleable splint on her right long finger to calculate optimum position for PIP on the left.

Figure 6 (a) Postarthritic ankylosis of the PIP joint of the left long finger producing a fixed swan-neck deformity. (b) The patient continues to play with difficulty using atypical fingering.

accurately measured and reproduced at the time of surgery. There are no norms and the players themselves can best decide the most suitable compromise position by using a small tempo-rary malleable splint to experiment (Fig. 8). If the musician has already adopted a slightly unusual fingering to accommodate a stiffened joint, and this joint has subsequently ankylosed in a non-functional position, one should attempt to gain the original compromised but functional position, rather than striving for 'normality'.

The case demonstrated (Figs 6–13) is an excel-lent illustration of the complexity and precision in preoperative planning for arthrodesis. This partic-ular young violinist had progressively developed ankylosis of the proximal interphalangeal (PIP) joint of her left (fingering) long finger secondary to an isolated brief polyarthropathy of unknown aetiology occurring when she was a teenager. She continued as a professional violinist using trick fingering to accommodate the swan-neck deformity. But as complete ankylosis developed, this became increasingly difficult. Because the joint was rigid, a trial position could not be tested on the left hand. Her fingering was unconven-tional and therefore her musical colleagues could not act as guinea pigs. Fortunately, talented as she is, she was able to play in the reversed position and a malleable trial splint was applied

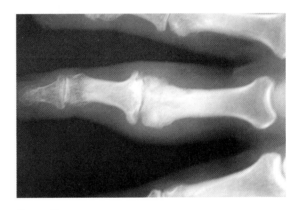

Figure 7

X-ray of PIP joint of left long finger.

to her right long finger! It was concluded that 50° of flexion was the optimum compromise position. This position was reproduced exactly at the time of surgery and a tension band compres-sion arthrodesis performed.

More commonly the distal joint is involved. By a similar process the ideal playing position can

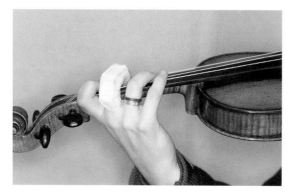

Figure 8

Trial splintage using a malleable splint on her right long finger (the left was too stiff to splint) to obtain the optimal angle for surgical arthrodesis.

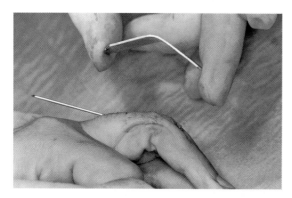

Figure 9

Malleable splint at surgery being used as a template for positioning of the arthrodesis.

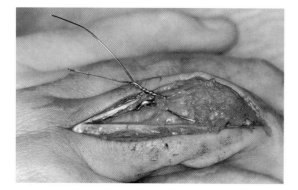

Figure 10

Tension band arthrodesis completed without interference on the extensor mechanism.

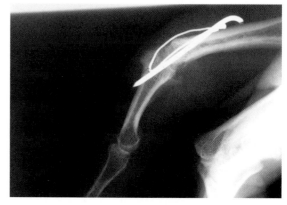

a

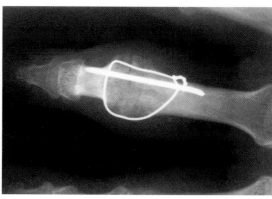

b

Figure 11

(a, b) Lateral and anteroposterior X-ray of compression arthrodesis.

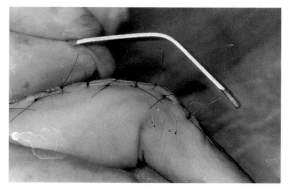

Figure 12

Re-check of final position of digit.

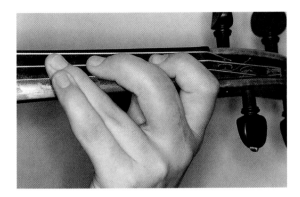

Figure 13

Return to instrument at 6 weeks.

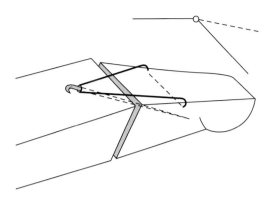

Figure 14

Tension band arthrodesis of the DIP joint. Note the use of a single k-wire and a △ (triangular) tension band to reduce the bulk of metal dorsally. Also note precise location of the distal tip of the k-wire penetrating but not protruding beyond the distal cortex.

be found (see Chapter 10, secondary reconstruction by surgical releases and skin grafting). The technique of DIP tension band arthrodesis is shown (Fig. 14). One strives for an early return to limited playing with these patients. The tension band technique certainly facilitates this and, apart from the left hand in string players and guitarists, limited playing can usually be allowed from the third week. The placement of the k-wire tip is critical in this context. It should penetrate the distal cortex but should not protrude into the pulp, which would cause great tenderness.

Arthrodesis of the distal joint is reliable in providing stability, strength and a specific position. Arthroplasty using one of the manufactured silastic implants gives excellent relief of pain and will provide some degree of mobility. However, it may not provide the required stability in any given situation, nor the required strength. The implant itself may fracture under the continuous loading one sees in a string player's left fingering hand. But in certain circumstances, an implant rather than arthrodesis would be the procedure of choice, particularly in the PIP joints of the more ulnar fingers where some mobility may be critical, or in the CMC joint which is inherently more stable, provided adequate ligament reconstruction is performed

at the time of replacement arthroplasty, and where again mobility may be critical.

In summary, osteoarthritis of one or more of the finger joints in a musician need not be the end to a playing career. By meticulously analysing the functional needs of the musician and the role that each joint plays in playing and by judicious use of appropriate splintage, conservative treatment or localized surgical intervention, one can in fact provide functioning, stable, painless joints even in the face of quite widespread generalized disease.

Rotator cuff

Christopher B Wynn Parry

Rotator cuff lesions are common particularly in string players. The condition is commoner in the bowing arm, although it is seen also in the violinist's left arm through static hold of the instrument. Cellists are not infrequently involved. Conductors who have been particularly vigorous in the use of their arms, employing for instance the Bernstein approach rather than the Reiner or Adrian Boult approach, may towards the end of their career sustain wear of their rotator cuff.

Care must be taken in the excessive use of steroid injections. We have seen many instrumentalists and conductors who have had regular and frequent injections of steroid into their rotator cuff to tide them through performances and the result has in some cases been disastrous, with total destruction of the rotator cuff requiring major surgery to restore function. Prevention is by far the best management, and an overhaul of technique is necessary, with methods of supporting the instrument and practice techniques being studied carefully.

Thoracic spine

The thoracic spine is a frequent source of symptoms causing aching pain across the back of the shoulders and into the neck. As a result of an abnormal posture adopted to minimize symptoms, pain may develop down the arm and secondary rotator cuff lesions may develop. This is a notoriously difficult area and expert physiotherapy assessment is essential, with careful attention to playing and practice techniques and the use of supports and harnesses.

Tennis elbow

Ian Winspur

The term 'tennis elbow' is a misnomer, for only a minority of sufferers have ever played tennis. It is, however, a common condition not only occurring in patients involved in heavy manual work, but also in those in clerical and professional work (Narakas and Bonnard 1991). Indeed, mild tennis elbow is not uncommon among musicians, although the exact pathophysiology of the condition in musicians may not be immediately obvious. The condition is also called 'lateral epicondylitis'. This also is a misnomer, for the epicondyle per se is not usually involved, but more the tendons of the common extensor origins distal to the epicondyle, particularly the tendinous origin of extensor carpi radialis brevis (ECRB). Surgical exploration of this area in

sufferers of tennis elbow has demonstrated small granulating tears on the undersurface of ECRB, non-healing larger tears and ruptures covered with frank granulation tissue and also chronic chondroid or calcific degeneration in the tendon. Occasionally underlying pathology of the radial head has also been identified, and more distal exploration has demonstrated compression of the radial nerve under fibrous bands on the undersurface of ECRB or by vascular arcades and a fibrous muscular rim as the deep branch of the nerve dives beneath supinator. However, the eponym 'tennis elbow', coined over a century ago, is here to stay.

Tennis elbow is more common in patients between 40 and 55 years of age. It presents as an aching around the lateral aspect of the elbow with intermittent severe discomfort associated with any activity requiring wrist and sometimes finger extension. Such activities as carrying suitcases, heavy bags or instrument cases (activities which in fact consume an inordinate amount of most musicians' day), produce extreme discomfort localized over the lateral epicondyle. Occasionally the onset of symptoms can be attributed to a specific instance of suddenly lifting a heavy object, or to a specific injury, usually a blow on the outer aspect of the elbow, but in the majority of cases no such incident can be identified. So-called cumulative trauma has been incriminated but the evidence is not scientific. Chronic light repetitive motion has also been incriminated and indeed accepted in the United States as a cause. However, again the evidence is unscientific and part of the acceptance in the US is due to the language of American Workman's Compensation legislation in which the issue of true causation is minimized. Indeed, in the musician population, if sustained repetitive light injury were actually a significant causative factor one would expect a much higher incidence of the more severe forms of tennis elbow. The symptoms of even mild tennis elbow can be so disruptive and distressing that musicians may find themselves temporarily completely unable to play and certainly incapable of managing the other duties involved in their daily routine, particularly the carrying of bags, briefcases and musical instruments. Additional symptoms beyond those localized around the elbow may develop as the musician continues to play and to spare the affected part.

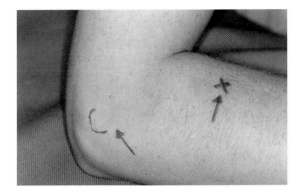

Figure 15

Arrows indicate the lateral epicondyle and the point of maximum tenderness (x) in radial tunnel syndrome.

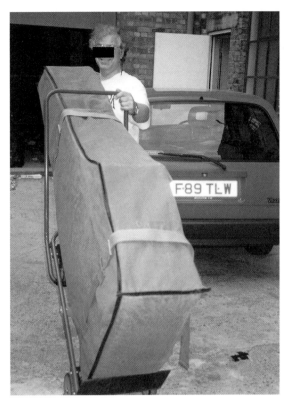

Figure 16

Use of wheels on a heavy instrument case (here a harpsichord) to minimize manhandling and the chances of developing tennis elbow (by courtesy of Michael Freyham).

So shoulder and neck pains and even contralateral shoulder pain may all develop in the musician from unilateral tennis elbow. When the condition is well established, secondary irritation of the radial nerve in the adjacent forearm may produce more diffuse distal symptoms, with distal forearm aching and distal dysaesthesia.

The diagnosis of the condition is made on clinical grounds – typical symptoms in association with very localized tenderness over or just distal to the lateral epicondyle. Provocative testing of wrist and finger extension will reproduce the pain. The most important but sometimes related condition to exclude is radial tunnel syndrome (Crawford 1984), or irritation or entrapment of the radial nerve adjacent to the elbow. Radial tunnel syndrome is seen in 5–10% of cases of tennis elbow and the relationship of the two conditions may be closely intertwined. The cardinal sign of radial tunnel syndrome is pain on deep palpation of the radial nerve deep to the common extensor wad, i.e. tenderness more distal on the forearm than seen in true tennis elbow (Fig. 15). Provocative testing of ECRB will reproduce symptoms in both conditions and the well-touted resisted long finger extensor test is also unreliable. Other sources of elbow pain arising from the elbow joint itself should also be excluded and X-rays of the elbow joint should always be obtained before dismissing this as the source of the pain.

Fortunately, the majority of patients suffering mild to moderate tennis elbow will recover spontaneously or with the help of steroid injections into the inflamed and damaged area. However, recovery is slow and can only be achieved if all activities producing symptoms are curtailed for at least a month to 6 weeks following resolution of symptoms either spontaneously or following injection. This is difficult for musicians.

Conservative treatment is to be preferred. This must consist of a careful analysis of mechanical factors involved both in playing and outside playing and modifications made thereto. Wheels can be added to heavy instrument cases (Fig. 16) and shoulder straps to lighter instrument cases and briefcases, and recreational travel can be curtailed or modified. A firm strap applied over the proximal forearm muscle mass may provide good symptomatic relief until the condition has settled. Oral NSAIDs may also give symptomatic relief as too may local NSAID ointment. Physical modalities such as deep direct massage over the injured area and gentle conditioning may also be of benefit and allow healing of the lesion. In chronic cases, where the condition has remained unchanged for many months despite repeated steroid injections, the first consideration is exclusion of other causes, particularly radial tunnel syndrome. This can only be done by careful clinical examination as electrodiagnostic testing is unreliable in this situation. Secondly, recurrent or repeated injury must also be ruled out or addressed. If indeed the condition is chronic and disabling then one may have to resort to a surgical solution. This is rare in our experience, although tennis elbow itself is not. The surgical results, which are unpredictable even in the less physically taxed general population, are likely also to be unpredictable in the musician. Nevertheless, if the musician's career is in jeopardy, then one may have little choice but surgery.

Multiple surgical techniques have been described. We have no personal experience of tennis elbow releases on professional musicians, nor have we been able to locate anyone who does. In principle, the operation of choice would be both predictable and straightforward, with the minimum of postoperative morbidity allowing an early return to playing. Other authors' experience of ECRB release and lengthening and its complications in sportsmen would not indicate this to be an appropriate treatment for musicians, however. The straightforward approach of the resection of involved tissue, epicondylar shaving and repair of the extensor origin (Froimson 1993), which has worked well in our experience in many non-musicians, would be the logical choice. If clear preoperative clinical signs of coexistent radial tunnel syndrome are present, then obviously the neural component must also be addressed. We have seen many non-musicians recover completely and rapidly when both the radial nerve and the tendon origins of the lateral epicondyle have been treated simultaneously, but I believe one must be sceptical about the likelihood of a professional musician returning to his full career after surgery of this nature.

The musculotendinous origins on the medial epicondyle can be the site of similar pathology producing similar symptoms on the inner aspect of the elbow (golfer's elbow). This is less common and more resistant to treatment than tennis elbow but is managed along exactly the same lines.

In summary, mild tennis elbow – for want of a better name – is not uncommon among musicians. The diagnosis must be made accurately on clinical grounds. The condition will normally settle with conservative care but resolution is slow. If one is forced to consider surgery, the results in musicians should be considered unpredictable at best.

Tendonitis

Ian Winspur

The word 'tendonitis' means inflammation of a tendon. However, its usage in a clinical setting is much wider and at times inappropriate. Tendonitis is acknowledged as a work-related disorder, even under the strict criteria of British prescribed industrial diseases (Harrington 1992), and for this reason the term seems to be used as a convenient label for many unrelated painful conditions in the arm. It is this misuse of the term which causes many otherwise conscientious and wise physicians to recoil and to avoid using the term at all, even in clinical situations where quite clearly sufficient signs are present to describe a specific tendon or group of tendons as being clinically inflamed. Indeed, to allow the diagnosis of tendonitis, a specific tendon or group of tendons must be swollen, tender, nodular and painful to move, and be associated with overlying bruising, erythema or crepitus (peritendonitis crepitans). And it is only when these specific clinical signs are present that the term may be used in referring to a musician's hand or arm. Both flexor or extensor tendons can be involved, seldom simultaneously. Tendons when running in sheaths or around pulleys or under retinacula are surrounded by thin mobile sheets of tissue or tenosynovium which can become swollen and tender (tenosynovitis). This term should only be used when such a clinical situation exists. It should not be used as a general term for diffuse hand or arm pain.

True inflammation can occur to tendons in generalized inflammatory diseases such as rheumatoid arthritis. However, much more frequently clinical tendonitis occurs in the absence of such diseases and often without any obvious precipitant. Histologically, inflammatory cells are seldom seen in the so-called inflamed tendons or surrounding tenosynovial tissue. Sometimes tendonitis does develop or appear as an apparent response to some unusual or unaccustomed mechanical loading or strain or activity. The exact correlation between clinical tendonitis and mechanical factors is hotly debated at the present time. Although so-called repetitive strain has been incriminated and indeed administratively accepted in the USA as a potent cause of tendonitis, no direct cause and effect has ever been scientifically demonstrated between tendonitis and repetitive light loading. If any group of people repetitively load specific isolated tendons, it is musicians, and yet true clinical tendonitis is surprisingly unusual in this group and more often relates more to extracurricular DIY (home improvements) activities or sport than to musical endeavours. But it would be incorrect completely to discount mechanical factors, for indeed one of the commonest clearly identified forms of tendonitis – de Quervain's tendonitis, which affects the tendons of the first extensor compartment as they run in a separate tight compartment over the radial border of the wrist – is very commonly seen in young mothers constantly handling small children. It is not only seen in biological mothers, but also in adoptive mothers and occasionally in young fathers. De Quervain's tendonitis has also been seen in the wrists of young female, non-nursing bassoon players, presumably from a similar mechanism while playing. The only common element in these groups is the unaccustomed, constant abnormal loading of the first extensor tendons with the wrist in a slightly abnormal position when handling a small child. It is also observed, but not scientifically proven, that the combination of frequent power gripping on an instrument or tool which simultaneously exerts direct pressure over the proximal pulley of the flexor tendon sheaths (secateurs, manual crimping

tools, pliers or gymnastic grip strengthening equipment) also seems to favour the development of trigger fingers. And indeed this has been seen in music students taking the lessons on physical fitness to heart and who overindulge in this particular method of attempting to increase forearm and intrinsic hand strength (personal communication, Prof. U. Büchler).

Clinical presentation

The clinical diagnosis of tendonitis requires the physical signs of swelling, tenderness and pain on passive movement to be present on a specific tendon (Lister 1993a). Additional signs which may be present are bruising, crepitus, redness, skin swelling and triggering. Triggering only occurs when the swollen tendon has to run into a confined space, in a separate compartment or into a tendon sheath under a tight pulley (trigger finger), when the swollen part of the tendon catches and snaps as it passes to and fro entering into the constricted area. Triggering is therefore only seen when certain specific tendons are involved in very localized and specific areas. Sites of triggering can be:

- Flexor tendons in the palm or digit – classic trigger finger
- First extensor compartment – de Quervain's tendonitis (unusual)
- Thumb extensor tendon – triggers as it rounds Lister's tubercle (rare)
- Extensor tendons on the dorsum of the wrist – interception syndrome where the first and second compartment extensor tendons cross each other immediately proximal to the wrist joints.

The clinical examination of tendons requires precise knowledge of the exact anatomical course of the tendon in question (Tubiana et al 1996). The tendon is then placed under tension by resisting the active motion of that tendon, and with this manoeuvre the tendon in question can be easily palpated (Finkelstein's test for de Quervain's tendonitis is an example of this manoeuvre) (Fig. 17). This test is a provocative test of the inflamed tendons of the first extensor compartment present in de Quervain's tendonitis.

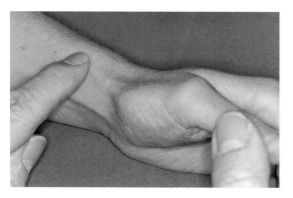

Figure 17

Modification of Finkelstein's test whereby the inflamed first extensor compartment tendons are provoked and palpated.

The test as originally described resisting radial deviation and abduction of the thumb with the wrist ulnarly deviated is confusing, as it may also provoke pain arising from both the basal joint of the thumb and the radial aspect of the wrist joint. The test is better performed as shown in Fig. 17, where the specific tendons involved are provoked, but are also highlighted and can be directly palpated. Not only should the patient's pain be reproduced by this manoeuvre, but the tendons and tendon sheath should feel thickened and tender. When these signs are not present the diagnosis of tendonitis cannot be made. When vague aching and tender areas in muscles are the only signs, tendonitis does not exist! Peripheral nerves adjacent to inflamed tendons can be transiently influenced – presumably on the basis of local oedema (Fig. 18). So, commonly, patients will also complain of some transient, altered sensibility or numbness in adjacent areas. For instance patients with de Quervain's tendonitis will sometimes complain of dysaesthesia over the radial dorsal aspects of the wrists. Patients with flexor tenosynovitis of the digit will similarly complain of transient numbness in that digit and pianists with flexor tenosynovitis of the wrist may also complain of transient dysaesthesia in the distribution of the median nerve. These patients *are not* suffering from one of the compression

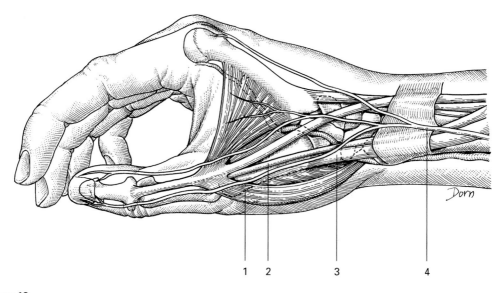

Figure 18

Anatomy of the first extensor compartment and radial border of the wrist. Note the tendons of abductor pollicis brevis, extensor pollicis brevis and abductor pollicis longus (1, 2, 3) running under a tight retinaculum over the radial styloid. Note the close proximity of the sensory branch of the radial nerve (4). (From Tubiana et al 1990.)

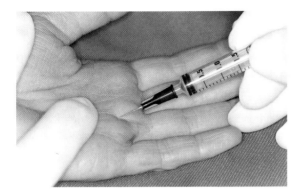

Figure 19

Site of injection of flexor tendon sheath for classic trigger fingers. Note: palpating digit of free hand; short fine needle; oblique direction of entry.

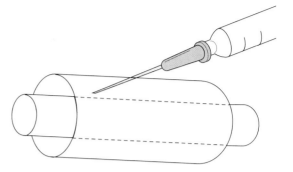

Figure 20

Diagrammatic representation of tendon sheath injection showing how an oblique entry into the tendon sheath increases the chances of finding the potential space between tendon and sheath into which the steroid should be injected (by courtesy of L. Murray RGN).

neuropathies. Nerve conduction tests will be normal.

Which musicians suffer tendonitis? Any musician when indulging in unaccustomed DIY (home improvements) is vulnerable, and home decoration involving paint-stripping and prolonged manual sanding is notorious for precipitating classic acute severe peritendonitis crepitans. Under normal circumstances, musicians playing their accustomed instruments in their ordinary and unextended fashion will not develop tendonitis. However, pianists particularly when indulging in extended practice of very complicated and technically demanding pieces are vulnerable and do present with isolated swollen, tender flexor tendons in either hand or in either wrist. Violinists similarly when playing difficult pieces with extensive vibrato do develop tender swollen tendons, particularly of the long and ring fingers of the left hand, and so do guitarists.

Treatment

Tendons are living self-repairing structures and tendonitis is therefore a self-limiting condition and should heal spontaneously. However, it can be extremely painful and requires vigorous supportive measures in the acute phase. This is one of the very few occasions when absolute rest for

musicians for 24–48 hours may be indicated. Additionally, ice, elevation and NSAIDs may help. When the condition is less acute, particularly when involving tendons running in sheaths, local steroid injections into the tendon sheath can be of great value (McGrath 1984). One injection will usually produce cure but the technique of injection is very important (Fig. 19). A mixture of non-absorbable steroid and local anaesthetic is used. This reduces the discomfort from the injection and also dilutes the suspension to allow freer flow of the particulate matter through the very fine needles used. Usually a short 26 or 28 gauge needle is used. The needle is inserted at a very oblique angle as this quite markedly increases the chances of entering the very narrow potential space between the tendon and the sheath (Fig. 20). The steroid should neither be injected directly into the tendon nor injected outside the sheath. If the needle is inserted vertically to the tendon sheath, then one of these sites of injection is guaranteed. Using lack of resistance as a gauge to the presence of the needle in the tendon sheath but not in the tendon, 2 ml of the mixture is injected. While injecting, one should be palpating the area of the injection and with the free hand one should feel a 'sausage' of distended tissues spreading along the tendon sheath in question if the injection has been properly placed (Fig. 21).

When the situation is truly chronic, the physical modalities of heat, ultrasound and deep massage

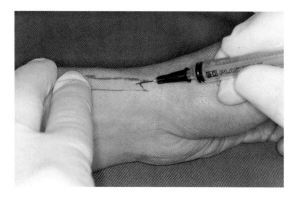

Figure 21

Injection of first extensor compartment.

of swelling and tenderness over specific tendons. This situation is less common in musicians than one would imagine. These clinical signs may be associated with symptoms of triggering or of dysaesthesia in adjacent nerves. The treatment for tendonitis should in general be conservative. Playing may need to be reduced but a degree of practice playing must be maintained. In a very few specific circumstances, when conservative care has failed, surgical decompression may be warranted.

Swellings

Ian Winspur

Hand infections are very rare in musicians. Apart from this, however, they suffer the same coincidental medical conditions as the general public. Hence the common benign tumours (ganglions etc.) are commonly seen among musicians. Malignant tumours, rare in the general population, are only very occasionally encountered in the much smaller, selected population of musicians. In fact, they are so rare that they are not worth considering in this context. In any case, their management is dictated by the medical and surgical requirements of the malignant tumour rather than the musician's unique needs. Similarly, premalignant tumours (skin cancers etc.) (Fleegler 1987) should also be managed along standard lines, the patient's occupation notwithstanding.

In our experience, ganglions and giant cell tumours are the commonest swellings encountered. Of over 600 musicians attending an upper extremity clinic, 2% were diagnosed as having

are of great help. Playing should be limited but not curtailed and practice sessions should be restricted to no longer than 5–10 minutes per session, with three to four sessions per day. As the condition eases the amount of playing should be steadily increased. Full rehearsal should not be resumed, however, until the patient has conditioned himself to that level and duration of playing in practice. The resolution of tendonitis is frustratingly slow and many patients remain intermittently symptomatic for 12–18 months – a disaster for the professional musician. Prevention is therefore much better than cure. Surgery has little place to play in the treatment of tendonitis in musicians even when triggering is occurring. It is only when all other modalities of treatment have failed, particularly if there remains frank triggering, that surgery should be contemplated. Indeed, in treating de Quervain's tendonitis, in patients playing certain instruments, particularly the violin where both wrists are held for long periods in abnormally flexed and radially deviated positions, there is such grave danger of the extensor tendons dislocating volarly following the release of the retinaculum (White and Weiland 1984) that surgical release in these circumstances should probably not be performed. In general, surgical release should only be considered in musicians as a last resort.

In summary, the diagnosis of tendonitis should only be made when there are clear clinical signs

Table 1 Diagnosis in 34 professional musicians undergoing hand surgery

Dupuytren's contracture	8	23.5%
Tumours (6 ganglions, 2 giant cell tumours)	8	23.5%
Trauma	7	20%
Carpal tunnel syndrome	5	15%
Osteoarthritis (arthrodesis)	3	9%
Cubital tunnel syndrome	2	6%
Osteoarthritis (synovectomy)	1	3%
	34	

ganglions. However, in our personal experience of professional musicians undergoing surgery, 8 out of 34 (23.5%) had operations for ganglions or giant cell tumours (see Table 1). This discrepancy results from the fact that patients had been referred with ganglions from outside the clinic system, and that ganglions which would have been to all intents and purposes asymptomatic or trouble-free in the general population have been referred with subtle difficulties requiring operative treatment. Giant cell tumours are significant because of their occurrence in the younger patient and because of their location, usually adjacent to critical tactile areas. Metacarpal bosses are significant because of the subtle disruption they can cause the finely balanced movements of the musician. Other benign tumours occur: lymphomas, sebaceous cysts, enchondromas and small vascular abnormalities – and they are handled in the conventional way. If excisional biopsy is felt to be appropriate, great care must be taken in the location of the skin incisions when dealing with these lesions. The patients should also be encouraged to return to limited playing at the earliest moment.

Digital neuromas also occur in discrete critical areas specific to various instruments (see Chapter 9). Surgery is contraindicated in the management of these lesions. Resolution can normally be achieved by suitable modification of the instrument or the musician's technique and can be speeded up by a perineural steroid injection.

Wrist ganglions

Dorsal wrist ganglions (Fig. 22) are the most commonly encountered, but volar wrist ganglions are also seen. Despite the cavalier attitude taken by doctors to ganglions in the general population, they can in fact produce symptoms. This is particularly true when they are arising and stretching periarticular tissues, when a dull aching pain is often produced. However, sometimes these symptoms remain even after the ganglion has ceased to increase in size. When static in size but symptomatic, they can cause loss of extreme wrist flexion associated with discomfort. They can also cause

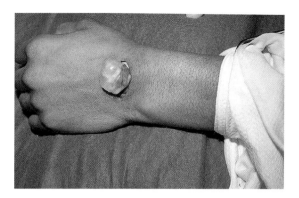

Figure 22

Typical dorsal wrist ganglion during surgical removal (by courtesy of Dr D Phelps).

inflammation of adjacent extensor tendons due to simple mechanical interference or irritation of the adjacent tendons – extensor tendonitis. These symptoms are seldom severe enough in the general population to warrant action. However, in the musician, particularly if the playing position requires extreme left wrist flexion or the ganglion is clearly causing extensive tendonitis with prolonged playing, action needs to be taken. There is still a place for the heavy book, although family Bibles seem no longer to exist. There is also a place for aspiration and steroid injection: despite the fact that recurrence rate is high, this is particularly appropriate in the active professional musician developing a symptomatic ganglion but requiring to continue playing. If all else fails, then surgical removal is indicated by the standard techniques. This is done through a transverse incision on the dorsum of the wrist and with careful dissection of the stalk of the ganglion directly down to the wrist joint and removal of a tiny window of the joint capsule with the base of the lesion. The musician has to be guided on recovery times, which will depend upon the instrument involved. In our experience, return to full playing when the playing is with the wrist extended and wrist movement is not critical (brass players) has been 2 weeks. However, in patients in whom extreme wrist flexion is required (violinists) or in whom free movement of the wrist is required (pianists) the average time to full playing, despite an early return to the instrument somewhere between 2 and 3 weeks following surgery, has been 6–8 weeks. The musician should also be warned of the known incidence of recurrence at somewhere around 5%.

Flexor sheath ganglions

Our experience has been that these lesions are remarkably common in drummers and tympanists, but also occur in other instrumentalists. Many musicians do not have symptoms from these lesions and no action needs to be taken once the diagnosis is established. However, particularly in drummers, certain symptoms occur – slight discomfort, slightly annoying and irritating mechanical interference by the small ganglion with the gripping of the drumstick, sufficient to upset the drummer's technique. Indeed, this may be enough to unbalance the musician's techniques in such a way that their presenting symptoms may not be obviously linked to the hand but may be diffuse symptoms of aching in the arm, shoulder and neck. It is only after careful searching that the true source of the problem is highlighted. When these flexor sheath ganglions are causing symptoms, even if diffuse and distant from the site of the lesion, it has been our experience that surgical removal performed through the standard short palmar or digitopalmar incisions, with extreme care taken of the digital nerves, has been dramatically effective. The patients have returned to playing at a very early point, usually with stitches in place, and have returned to full playing in 10–14 days.

Giant cell tumours

Giant cell tumours (Fig. 23), otherwise known as villonodular synovitis and incorrectly known as xanthomas (Lister 1993b), do occur in younger patients and occur in critical areas adjacent to the flexor surfaces or pulp surfaces of the digits. Our personal experience indicates that they represent 30% of professional musician patients undergoing surgery for removal of swellings and tumours. Of the two musician patients we have

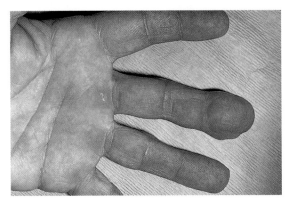

Figure 23

Typical giant cell tumour arising from the PIP joint and involving the pulp of the digit (by courtesy of Dr D Phelps).

treated, one, a jazz guitarist, had a lesion involving the central pulp of the right thumb, and the other, a young violinist, had a lesion involving the radial border of the pulp of the right index finger. These tumours are not malignant, but if left unattended, they steadily increase in size, wrap around flexor and extensor tendons spreading both volarly and dorsally in the digit and cause bony changes due to compression (Glowacki and Weiss 1995). Their removal requires meticulous dissection (Fig. 24) for the rate of recurrence, due to either macro- or microscopically incomplete excision, can be as high as 50%. The siting of incisions is obviously critical because good exposure is required, but the scar cannot violate a critical tactile area. Hence, in the case of the bowing right index finger of a young violinist, a mid-lateral approach was used along the radial border of the distal digit, but the incision was moved 2 mm dorsally to avoid the area noted preoperatively to be in direct contact with the bow. The so-called open book incision (mid-lateral with transverse dorsal and volar extensions) should be avoided. The vascularity of the flaps is questionable and the disruption to cutaneous sensibility is unacceptable. Lesions involving the pulp of digits, for instance in the right thumb pulp of the guitarist mentioned earlier, should be approached directly with longitudinal incisions in the axis of the digit passing

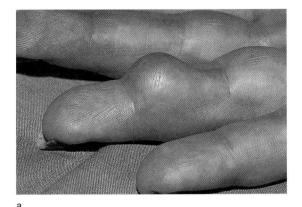

a

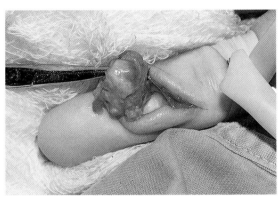

b

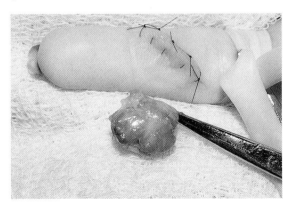

c

Figure 24

(a, b, c) Intraoperative photographs of giant cell tumour embracing flexor tendon (by courtesy of Dr D Phelps).

vertically and directly through the pulp to the lesion. This approach interferes least with the terminal branches of the digital nerves, causes little scarring and in our experience with musicians and non-musicians causes the least disruption to the fine tactile sensitivity of the pulp. Fish mouth incisions or indirect approaches through radial or ulnar incisions cause significant sensory disturbance and scarring and should be avoided. A meticulous excision much reduces the chance of recurrence but should the lesion recur, recision via the same incision with suitable extension should be performed.

Metacarpal bosses

A prominence at the base of the second and third metacarpals and adjacent carpal bones at the insertion of the radial wrist extensors is a common finding and can seldom be credited with the symptoms claimed. However, some musician patients have complaints very suggestive of an irritative extensor tendonitis and have been cured by excision or certain smoothing of the bony prominence in that area. Nevertheless, one must be wary of this presentation and surgery should only be performed as a final resort. However, in two of our musician patients, both young female string players complaining of burning pain on the dorsum of their hand and wrist, on examination while playing there was clear evidence of dislocation of the extensor tendons over the bony prominence (Fig. 25). This was only demonstrable while playing with the wrist in the extreme flexed position and only involved the tendons to the index finger in a specific manoeuvre. One patient, a senior music student, was unable to play, but her symptoms have completely alleviated and she has returned to full performance following excision of the metacarpal boss. The second patient has not had surgery and has been lost to follow-up.

We therefore believe that if a metacarpal boss is present and there are clear signs of impingement or dislocation of an extensor tendon, which itself is thickened and tender, indications exist for removal or smoothing of the bony lesion.

In summary, basic medical and surgical principles apply to the management of swellings in the musician's hand. In benign lesions a conservative

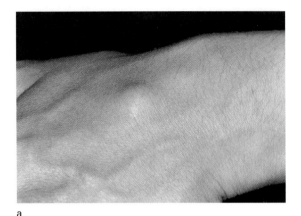
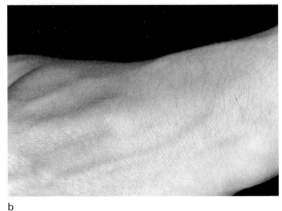

a   b

Figure 25

Dislocation of extensor tendon over metacarpal boss in a 23-year-old female. (a) Wrist in ulnar deviation highlighting the metacarpal boss with the index extensor tendons lying ulnar. (b) Radial deviation of the wrist with the index extensors now dislocated over the boss which lies between the index extensors and the common extensor to the long finger.

course is entirely appropriate, provided the doctor realizes that the somewhat unorthodox or possibly even bizarre symptoms claimed may indeed be due to such a lesion. When symptoms are present, even if present to a degree which in the general population would not require active intervention, if they are causing subtle difficulties in playing in the musician, then indeed active treatment is indicated and surgical excision may be appropriate. A full assessment of the patient's playing position and playing needs has to be made prior to such action and very careful siting of incisions must be planned. Additionally, the patient should be encouraged to return to limited playing at a very early point. When the patient will return to full playing will be determined by the nature of the instrument.

Hypermobility syndrome

Christopher B Wynn Parry

The condition known medically as the hyper-mobility syndrome (HMS) refers to the increased range of movement in certain joints, particularly the fingers, that laymen call double-jointed (Figs 26, 27). The term 'hyperlaxity', as suggested by

Bird, is probably more appropriate (Bird 1991). Some inherit shallow joints, or different degrees of tensile collagen in ligaments, for hyperlaxity or HMS is frequently inherited. The Indo-Asian races are naturally hypermobile. The extreme of the syndrome is the Ehlers–Danlos syndrome, where elasticity of collagen is widespread systemically and leads to cardiac, visual and other symptoms. This, however, is rare. Larsson (Larsson et al 1987) refers to the finding by Hippocrates that the Scythians showed an extremely high degree of hypermobility. The males had such lax joints that they were hardly able to pull a bow or hurl a javelin. He notes that present day Iyaggis are probably descendants of the Scythians and are extremely hypermobile.

Many authors have drawn attention to the relative frequency of HMS in musicians. Possibly they are self-selected, as the increase in range favours increased technical ability. Paganini and Rachmaninof and probably Liszt were all capable of remarkable flexibility of the fingers and thumb and wide spans allowing the playing of a twelfth with ease. HMS is particularly helpful in playing the guitar. The syndrome is commoner in females than males and has a peak incidence at 12–15 years and then tends slowly to decline. It is least manifest in the early morning and most in the afternoon. Tall, thin people are more likely

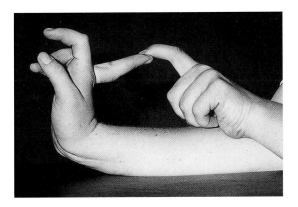

Figure 26

Passive dorsiflexion of the little finger beyond 90°.

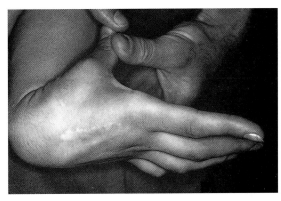

Figure 27

Passive apposition of the thumbs to the flexor aspects of the forearm.

to be hypermobile than short and stocky people. It has long been recognized that hypermobile people are more liable to sustain stretching injuries with sprains of joints, effusions and occasionally tendonitis. Diaz et al (1993) studied 675 male soldiers. Of these 67% showed no joint laxity, 25.5% showed two or three lax joints, while 7.5% showed four or more. The occurrence of musculoskeletal lesions during regimes of physical exertion was significantly higher in the lax and hyperlax individuals. What has recently become clear is that the HMS syndrome is associated with widespread generalized aches and pains in proximal and distal limb muscles, but also sometimes in the spine. Hudson (Hudson et al 1995) reported that 13.2% of patients with soft tissue rheumatism showed HMS in 378 consecutive rheumatology patients. In another series, 3.25% of females and 0.63% of males in 9275 new referrals to a rheumatology clinic showed HMS with symptoms. Rodney Grahame, writing in an editorial in 1993 in the *New England Journal of Medicine* (Grahame 1993a), points out that it is one of the most common disorders encountered in rheumatological and orthopaedic practice provided it is looked for. He comments that physicians are rarely alert to increased joint motion and explains why the benign joint hypermobility syndrome is commonly overlooked,

misdiagnosed and hence inappropriately treated, leading to much unnecessary suffering. He goes on to point out that the syndrome is not invariably generalized, but may exist in a small number of joints or even in a solitary joint. This pauciarticular hypermobility was more prevalent than the generalized variety. It is therefore most important that all musicians attending an upper limb clinic are screened for HMS. It may well explain the local problem of joint or tendon involvement but also the very diffuse pains in the upper limb that are common presenting symptoms in musicians in such clinics.

Larsson (Larsson et al 1993) however has pointed out that HMS is not necessarily related to symptoms. He interviewed 660 musicians about symptoms related to playing and he concluded that among musicians who play instruments requiring repetitive motion, hypermobility of joints such as the wrist and elbows may be an asset, whereas hypermobility of less frequently moved joints such as the knees and spine may be a liability and may cause pain after long periods of sitting. Five of the 96 (5%) musicians with hypermobility of the wrists, mostly players of the flute, violin or piano, had pain and stiffness in that region, whereas 100 of the 564 musicians (18%) without such hypermobility had symptoms. It is therefore clear that symptoms from hypermobility are not inevitable, but clearly if the joints are being misused, with for example inappropriate practice schedules or poor technique with the wrong instrument, then symptoms are likely.

Rodney Grahame, in a most useful review in *Topical Reviews/Reports on Rheumatic Diseases*, series II (Grahame 1993b), has tabulated the musculoskeletal manifestations. They include myalgia and arthralgia, which can often be troublesome; soft tissue lesions commonly seen in everyday practice but occurring with greater frequency, often arising from trauma or overuse, including tennis elbow, tendonitis, capsulitis and carpal tunnel syndrome. Among other articular manifestations were traumatic joint synovitis or tenosynovitis; chronic monoarticular arthropathy or polyarthritis, which may mimic other forms of arthritis, particularly rheumatoid and juvenile chronic arthritis; and recurrent dislocations or subluxation of the shoulder or metacarpopha-langeal joints. He points out that a common complaint of these patients is a feeling of the joint slipping in and out of place with or without pain.

It is possible that HMS can lead to premature osteoarthritis, but most probably only if the joints are subjected to repeated trauma such as in high jumpers or ballet dancers. Carter and Wilkinson's scoring system for the hypermobility syndrome (Table 2) has been widely accepted. We would add from our own extensive experience exces-sive internal rotation of the shoulder with the ability of the patient to touch the cervical spine above T1 (Fig. 28) and an increased rotation of the neck's ability to bring the chin beyond the shoulder in looking backwards. We have noted patients with painful shoulders whose range on the affected side is within normal limits, but whose unaffected site is clearly hypermobile; there is thus relative stiffness of the affected joint which can be relevant, particularly in string players, who need full mobility of the shoulder. It must be emphasized that hypermobility may be confined to one set of joints only, e.g. the fingers or the thumb, or even a solitary joint. The full house of Carter and Wilkinson (Carter and Wilkinson 1964) is less frequent and it is commoner for HMS to affect a few joints only.

Hall and his colleagues (Hall et al 1995) showed that proprioceptive acuity in the knee joints of hypermobile people was reduced and this suggests a mechanism whereby their joints

Table 2 Scoring system for the hypermobility syndrome

Passive dorsiflexion of the little finger beyond 90°	1 point for each hand = 2 points
Passive apposition of the thumbs to the flexor aspects of the forearm	1 point for each thumb = 2 points
Hyperextension of the elbows beyond 10°	1 point for each elbow = 2 points
Hyperextension of the knees beyond 10°	1 point for each knee = 2 points
Forward flexion of the trunk with knees straight so that the palms of the hand rest easily on the floor	1 point
Total	9 points

are vulnerable. This of course can be particularly important in the hands and wrists of instru-mentalists. Mallik et al (1994) showed impaired proprioceptive acuity with HMS at the proximal interphalangeal joints in particular.

Management

Tendonitis and joint sprains are treated in the usual manner with judicious rest, local or systemic anti-inflammatory preparations and steroid injections (in cases that do not respond). We strongly believe that the key to long-term successful management is the development of adequate strength and stamina of the muscles controlling the hypermobile joint or joints. We explain to our patients that it is a blessing for them to have an increased range of movement with its implications of technical ability and we cite Paganini and Rachmaninof, but we point out that they are likely to pay for this if they do not develop sufficient strength and stamina of the appropriate muscles that control such joints. A session or two with an experienced hand thera-pist is of great value; they are instructed on a home exercise programme which they must follow assiduously (see Chapter 11). It is an easy matter to adapt rubber bands and pencils on a desk to provide steadily increasing resistance to the interossei and lumbricals and the wrist and finger extensors. It is important to be specific and

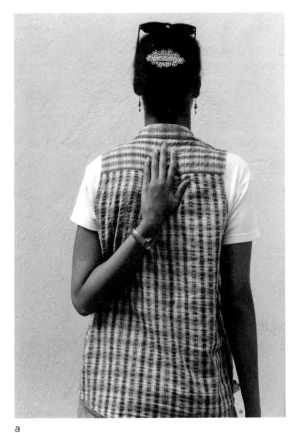
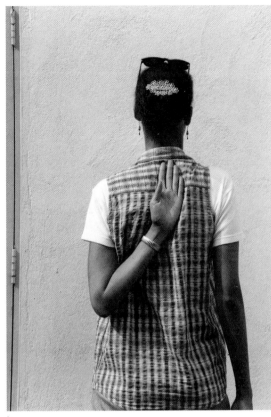

a

b

Figure 28

(a, b) A 23-year-old female violin student with 'lax joints' by conventional criteria; dramatic demonstration of overall hypermobility by this simple manoeuvre.

train the muscles surrounding the hypermobile joints and not give just a general physiotherapy programme for upper limb strengthening.

We invariably find that if hypermobility has been a significant factor in the generation of symptoms, such an intensive progressive course results in total relief of symptoms and renewed confidence in play. In the generalized form of hypermobility, an intensive progressive course of exercises to build up strength and stamina must be given to the whole body and this should include the spine, knees and hips, as well as the upper limbs. We prefer a skilled physiotherapist to supervise this, rather than suggesting the patients go to their local gymnasium. There is a

danger of patients overdoing it in the gymnasium; musicians, after all, are obsessional, dedicated people likely to seize the gym programme with enthusiasm, and may easily overdo it if not strictly controlled. Unsupervised weight-training or overenthusiastic regimes can easily lead to overstretching of already lax and vulnerable ligaments with resulting strains, sprains, effusions and tears of muscles. It is important to reassure patients that the condition is not serious and that with a sensible lifestyle and a regular exercise programme it should have no effect on their career.

We would like to emphasize again the vital importance of assessing every musician in a clinic for the hypermobility syndrome and this means being alert and examining all the joints of the upper limb, the spine and the knees and ankles.

References

Bird HA, Graham R (1991). *Rheumatic Complaints in the Performing Arts*. Reports on Rheumatic Diseases, May 1991, no. 18. Arthritis and Rheumatism Council: London.

Carter C, Wilkinson J (1964) Persistent joint laxity and congenital dislocation of the hip. *J Bone Joint Surg (Br)* **46**:40–5.

Crawford GP (1984) Radial tunnel syndrome (correspondence). *J Hand Surg* **9A**:451–2.

Diaz MA Estevez EC, Guijo PS (1993) Joint hyperlaxity and musculo-ligamentous lesions. *Br J Rheumatol* **32**:120–2.

Fleegler EJ (1987) Tumours involving the skin of the upper extremity. *Hand Clin* **3**:185–95.

Froimson A (1993) Tenosynovitis and tennis elbow. In: Green E, ed. *Operative Hand Surgery*, vol. 2 (3rd edn). Churchill Livingstone: New York: 1989–2006.

Glowacki KA, Weiss AP (1995) Giant cell tumours of tendon sheaths. *Hand Clin* **11**:245–53.

Grahame R (1993a) Joint hypermobility and the performing musicians. *N Engl J Med* **329**:1120–1.

Grahame R (1993b) Hypermobility syndrome. *Topical Reviews/Reports on Rheumatoid Diseases*, series II **25**:1–4.

Hall MG, Ferrell WR, Sturrock RD et al (1995) The effect of the hypermobility syndrome on knee joint proprioception. *Br J Rheumatol* **34**:121–5.

Harrington JM (1992) *Work-related Upper Limb Disorders*. DSS Report, HMSO: London.

Hudson N, Starr MR, Esdaile JM et al (1995) Diagnostic associations with hypermobility in new rheumatology referrals. *Br J Rheumatol* **34**:1157–61.

Lambert CM (1992) Hand and upper limb problems of instrumental musicians. *Br J Rheumatol* **31**:265–71.

Larsson L-G, Baum J, Mudholkar GS (1987) Hypermobility: features and differential incidence between the sexes. *Arthritis Rheum* **30**:1426–30.

Lederman RJ (1987) Thoracic outlet syndrome. *Med Probl Perform Artists* **2**:87–91.

Lister G (1993a) Inflammation. In: Lister G, ed. *The Hand: Diagnosis and Indications* (3rd edn). Churchill Livingstone: Edinburgh: 343–53.

Lister G (1993b) Swellings. In: Lister G, ed. *The Hand: Diagnosis and Indications* (3rd edn). Churchill Livingstone: Edinburgh: 435–40.

McGrath MH (1984) Local steroid therapy in the hand. *J Hand Surg* **9A**:915–21.

Mallik AK, Ferrell WR, McDonald AG et al (1994) Impaired proprioreceptive acuity at the PIP joint in patients with hypermobility syndrome. *Br J Rheumatol* **33**:631–7.

Narakas A, Bonnard C (1991) Epicondylalia: conservative and surgery treatment. In: Tubiana R, ed. *The Hand*, vol. 4. WB Saunders: Philadelphia: 835–57.

Nolan WB, Eaton RG (1989) Thumb problems of professional musicians. *Med Probl Perform Artists* **4**:20–2.

Norris R (1993) *The Musician's Survival Manual*. MNP Music Inc.: St Louis.

Palmieri JJ, Grand FM, Hay EL, Burk C (1987) Treatment of osteoarthritis of the hand. *Hand Clin* **3**:371–81.

Tubiana R, McCullough CJ, Masquelet AC (1990) *An Atlas of Surgical Exposures of the Upper Extremity*. Martin Dunitz/JB Lippincott: London/Philadelphia.

Tubiana R, Thomine JM, Mackin E (1996) Examination of the musculo-tendinous apparatus. In: Tubiana et al, eds. *Examination of the Hand and Wrist*. Martin Dunitz: London: 205–24.

White GM, Weiland AJ (1984) Symptomatic palmar tendon subluxation after surgical release for DeQuervain's tendonitis. *J Hand Surg* **9A**:704–6.

Wynn Parry CB, Stanley JK (1993) Synovectomy of the hand. *Br J Rheumatol* **32**:1089–95.

8
Dupuytren's contracture

Ian Winspur

Dupuytren's contracture is a hereditary condition occurring usually, but not exclusively, in males over 50 years of age and almost entirely of Northern European ancestry. It is in our experience very common among European orchestral players. It is uncommon among the Mediterranean races and virtually unknown in the Black and Oriental races. The afflicted develop nodules of fibrous tissue in the palm, which eventually form bands running into the finger. The ring finger is most commonly involved, then the little, the long, the index and the thumb. The rate of progression of the disease is extremely variable and may take many years, but in others digital bands and contracture develop in a few months. With progression of the bands into a digit, irrevocable flexion contracture will start to occur. Again, the rate is variable and may even be 'stop–go'. A small number of patients suffer a more active form of the disease – Dupuytren's diathesis – which occurs at a much younger age and spreads like wildfire to multiple digits. This is indeed a serious and difficult condition to treat, but is fortunately rare. A small number of patients suffering idiopathic epilepsy also suffer from Dupuytren's contracture and the faulty genes of the two conditions are known to be closely situated.

History and genetics (Elliott 1988)

The inheritance of Dupuytren's contracture is through an autosomal dominant gene of variable penetrance and herein lie continuing questions. For it is surprisingly rare for a sufferer to know of a living relative with the disease. In the United States of America, in spite of the massive immigration in the eighteenth and nineteenth centuries from Northern European countries, the condition is now much less common than currently in the countries of origin. The gene seems to be weakening in the USA. In Australia, however, Dupuytren's contracture is very common and Dupuytren's diathesis is seen remarkably frequently, the gene, probably having been introduced via a number of strongly afflicted Irish and Scottish families, remaining strong. With modern microbiology, DNA identification and gene mapping, studies are currently underway to clarify the inheritance.

Where did the faulty gene originally come from and when did it emerge? The condition was first described in 1614 in Basel by Felix Platter, but because it is so common in the Scandinavian countries, and those areas colonized by the Norse, it is assumed to have been introduced by the Vikings. However, early medical records of Anglo-Saxon monks on the east coast of England, which are detailed enough to allow clear identification of known dermatological and infectious diseases, give no mention of contractures of the hand. Yet on the Isle of Skye in the western islands of Scotland, an area colonized by the Norse, the MacCrimmon curse, a progressive contracture of the little fingers, has been known for centuries.

Bagpipers were held in high regard in the clan structure of Celtic Scotland. Indeed, they were ranked second only to the clan chieftain, who himself was selected by clan election rather than by accident of birth. This system was outlawed in 1747 with the defeat of the Jacobites by the English and the hazardous system of inherited aristocracy was imposed on the highland clans. Pre-eminent among bagpipe players were the MacCrimmons of Skye, who were pipers to the Chieftain of the Clan McCleod. Such was their reputation that a piping school was founded in

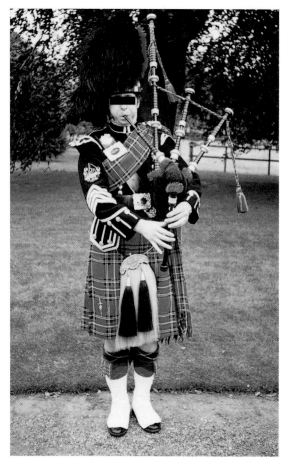

Figure 1

A Scottish bagpipe player: there is a high incidence of Dupuytren's contracture affecting the right little finger, making playing impossible.

Skye in the late fifteenth century and young talented pipers were sent from afar to hone their skills at this school for 2 to 3 years at a time. The school existed for many years until the Jacobite revolution and much of the surviving early pibroch music was from this school and was written by the MacCrimmons. However, the MacCrimmons were affected by a disease – a curse – which progressively bent the little finger. The little finger of the right hand is critical in playing the bagpipes (Fig. 1) and so the development of this affliction made

playing impossible. The family histories of those afflicted are lost in time and in the confusion following the crushing of the highland rebellion in 1745. However, even today many Scottish pipers become similarly afflicted by Dupuytren's contracture of the right little finger and it is still known as 'the curse of the MacCrimmons'.

Early confusion existed whether flexor tendons or palmar fascia were responsible for the contracture. It was Dupuytren, the senior surgeon at the Hôtel de Dieu in Paris who controversially, but firmly, in 1831 incriminated the palmar fascia. In fact an English surgeon, Henry Cline, had identified and incriminated the correct tissue in 1777, but his work was ignored even by his more famous and younger colleague, Astley Cooper, who in 1829 attributed the contracture to inflammation in both the tendon sheaths and the fascia. Hence, it is Dupuytren, the Frenchman, whose name rightly is attached to the condition.

Surgical rationale

Many musicians are male and over 50 years of age and therefore Dupuytren's contracture is one of the commonest afflictions and non-traumatic surgical conditions to be treated in musicians in the Western world. In our experience 30% of non-trauma cases in a series of 34 professional musicians undergoing operation were cases of Dupuytren's contracture. It is important to understand the rationale behind the modern surgical approach to Dupuytren's contracture because it allows one to formulate a sensible approach to the musicians suffering this condition. For in this group over-zealous surgery, with the complications of delayed wound healing, swelling and dense postoperative scarring, is as devastating as inadequate surgery with poor exposure, risk to nerves and vessels, inadequate release and early recurrence. Large series of cases, untreated and treated by the great variety of surgical techniques and postoperative regimes, are unfortunately not available. However, moderately large series of untreated cases and cases treated by the techniques of fasciotomy (simple division of the contracting band), conservative fasciectomy (where only abnormally involved tissue is excised) and radical fasciectomy (where both involved and uninvolved palmar fascia are excised) are documented (Winspur 1980). These series would confirm a number of basic points:

- The disease is chronic and recurring
- Recurrence is rapid following fasciotomy alone
- Recurrence is slowed following fasciectomy
- Postoperative complications are extremely high and recurrence not prevented following 'radical' fasciectomy
- Recurrence is slowed with the use of skin grafts.

Logically, it follows that the prerequisites of primary operation should be good exposure, healthy skin flaps and meticulous clearance of involved tissue. In recurrent disease, similar requirements need to be met, but additionally involved and scarred skin needs to be excised and skin grafts should be used both to overcome skin shortage and more importantly to slow the rate of recurrence.

At the time of writing, particularly since past experience has shown unacceptably high levels of complication from the more radical operations of wide fasciectomy of both involved and uninvolved tissue, most surgeons prefer conservative fasciectomies, but with a variety of surgical incisions, approaches and management of skin deficiencies.

From our perspective, Dupuytren's disease is a longitudinal disease; the contracting bands run longitudinally; the structures most likely to be damaged and which must be protected, the digital nerves, run longitudinally; the common sites of injury to digital nerves are at two levels, the metacarpo-phalangeal (MP) level proximally and at the distal end of the dissection distally. The significant early complication from surgery is delay in skin and wound healing, secondary either to haematoma or to poor skin vascularity associated with excessively thin or poorly designed flaps (Fig. 2). This diagrammatic representation demonstrates how the popular zigzag and curvy linear incisions criss-crossing the contracting band produce triangular or semi-elliptical flaps of poor vascularity based on the areas of thinned dermis dissected directly from the underlying contracting band. The 'Z'-plasty technique creates triangular flaps in which the

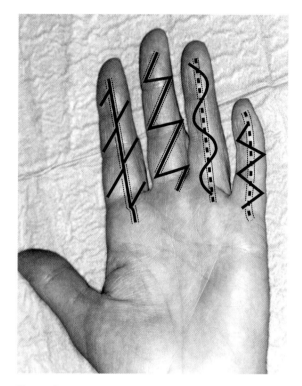

Figure 2

The skin incisions used in Dupuytren's contracture. The dotted areas represent areas of thinned dermis. Note the extensively compromised flaps produced by zigzag and curvilinear incisions on the little and ring fingers.

compromised areas involved one edge and not the base of the flaps and whose vascularity is healthy and derived from a normal subcutaneous base (Hueston 1984). We believe the Hueston approach (Hueston 1961) is certainly the preferred approach for primary Dupuytren's releases in musicians. Not only are the skin flaps healthier, but it also has the advantage of allowing additional skin to be advanced into the surgical areas and for the positioning of full-thickness flaps over exposed critical structures. If a skin shortage exists, small interpositional grafts can also be used, although this is usually only done in recurrent cases.

As discussed in Chapter 6, it is important that musicians should not be prevented from playing for a day longer than necessary. If one succeeds in obtaining primary wound healing following the release of Dupuytren's contracture, this period can ideally be kept as short as 5 days. The open palm technique (McCash 1964) has the advantage of minimizing postoperative haematoma formation, skin necrosis and wound dehiscence through tension. However, these complications can be prevented by proper technique in the closed methods and the open method has the great disadvantages of substantially prolonging postoperative hand swelling and the mechanical difficulties associated with the open wounds. These will prevent the ideal, very early return to limited playing for the musician as healing time and the complete resolution of swelling may take 2–3 weeks. For this reason alone, we do not believe the open palm technique is appropriate for the musician and stress again the use of the closed techniques (Table 1).

Recurrence of Dupuytren's contracture (assuming satisfactory initial release and absence of the so-called early 'reactivation') should be considered the norm. However, in most individuals recurrence is gradual and is over a 5- to 10-year period, and therefore surgical control can be considered to give fair respite and should enable the musician to continue his normal career. It is true that some individuals have a more aggressive form of the disease (Dupuytren's diathesis) with early widespread recurrence and development of plaques in ectopic and unusual sites. These people do have a strong tendency for early widespread postoperative recurrence, but fortunately the diathesis is rare and seems even rarer in musicians. In individuals with the Dupuytren's diathesis, replacement of involved skin by full-thickness skin grafts has been shown to halt the progress of the disease and this approach should be used. In primary Dupuytren's contracture, seldom is the skin extensively involved and seldom is one faced with true skin shortage, particularly when using a technique such as the multiple 'Z'-plasty where additional skin can be advanced without tension to overcome any slight skin shortage. However, when handling recurrent disease, matters are very different. Often the skin is extensively involved in the Dupuytren's process or may be densely scarred. This skin has to be sacrificed, thus creating a skin shortage. Complete resurfacing by full-thickness grafting,

sacrificing involved and normal skin, has been recommended (Logan et al 1985). However, in their series non-recurrence could not be guaranteed and the postoperative immobilization varied from 3 to 6 weeks – unacceptably long for a musician. Therefore radical resurfacing is not to be recommended, even in recurrent cases, in musicians.

In those individuals showing a tendency to recurrence, the rate of recurrence can be slowed by inserting *interpositional* full-thickness skin grafts. Techniques have been described where the recurrent bands are simply incised and interpositional grafts inserted (Gonzalez 1974). This is, in fact, technically difficult as the digital nerves are many times intimately bound to the longitudinal bands and scar and are in considerable jeopardy during a transverse release if they have not been previously identified and isolated. Obviously, this is not the situation to place oneself in when releasing a musician's hand and therefore we believe the correct approach in these circumstances is again a longitudinal approach with clear identification of all structures, the creation of well-vascularized thick 'Z'-plasty flaps in healthy skin, the sacrifice of any unhealthy scarred and involved skin and closure by a mixture of healthy triangular 'Z'-plasty flaps and full-thickness skin grafts interposed between these healthy flaps (Fig. 3). This technique combines the advantage of longitudinal exploration and 'Z'-plasty, and also the advantage of interposed full-thickness skin grafting. The healing time is much shorter than with complete resurfacing, the risks less and recurrence no greater, and this approach has served us well, particularly when dealing with very difficult and critical situations in the musician's hand with difficult, dense scar and recurrence.

Indications for surgery

In our experience, instrumentalists requiring wide span (pianists and bassoon players) (Fig. 4) in whom early contracting bands had developed between the web space of the little and ring fingers, restricting abduction of the little finger, can have considerable technical difficulty playing even in the absence of significant

Table 1 Analysis of professional musicians undergoing surgical release of Dupuytren's contracture 1986–1997 (all male)

Instrument	Age	Type of disease	Surgical technique	Weeks off instrument	Weeks to full performance	Follow up (years)
Piano	78	Primary	'Z'-plasty	3	8	7
Viola	50	Primary	'Z'-plasty	6	8	3
Bassoon	48	Recurrent	Intergraft*	2.5	6	3
Violin	47	Primary	'Z'-plasty	1.5	4	3
Violin	45	Primary	'Z'-plasty	1	3	2.5
Piano	72	Recurrent	Intergraft*	2	6	2
Guitar	33	Primary	Intergraft*	1	2	2
Trombone	65	Recurrent	Intergraft*	2	6	1
Average				2.4	5.3	3

*Local flaps with interpositional full-thickness grafts

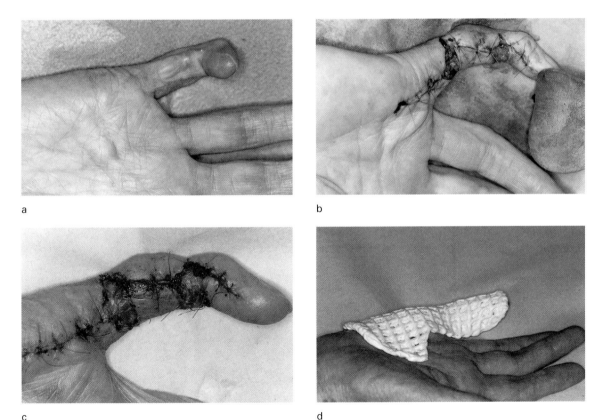

a b c d

Figure 3

(a) Severe recurrent Dupuytren's contracture of the little finger: the 90° distal interphalangeal contracture and 45° proximal interphalangeal contracture are incompatible with playing even a stringed instrument. (b) The existing scar and the skin involved in Dupuytren's contracture are released but healthy flaps are saved. (c) Wounds at 5 days with healing skin grafts between healthy flaps. (d) Postoperative splint.

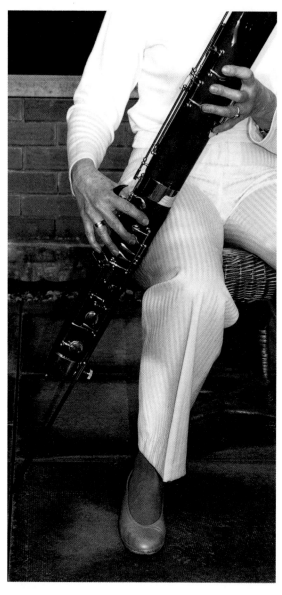

Figure 4

Position of hands on a bassoon. Note the wide span required in both hands in this female player with average-sized hands (by courtesy of Dr J Riley).

difficulty. Hence, standard indications for surgery do not apply to musicians, but Murphy's law does – if it is interfering with playing, surgical release is indicated, and if not leave well alone. When faced with a musician developing a troublesome Dupuytren's contracture, it should be stated from the outset that the condition is chronic and recurring and that the approach therefore is one of control, not cure. As such, the surgical approach should be careful and conservative, although it is recognized from experience that early recurrence in patients not suffering the severe form of the disease might possibly be related to incomplete removal of contracting tissue. Therefore, the surgical approach, particularly in the primary case, must also be thorough.

Our chosen techniques are longitudinal approach and multiple 'Z'-plasty closure for the primary case and for the recurrent case a similar approach but with excision of involved and scarred skin and interposition of short segmental full-thickness grafts (Fig. 3).

Postoperative care

The details of postoperative care are described in Chapter 11. But the principles are:

- High elevation and immobilization in a mildly compressive dressing and Plaster of Paris (POP) splint for 5 days
- Dressing and splint removal at 5 days, active daytime range of motion exercises, shadow playing + limited playing and finger exercises on the instrument 2–3 times a day for 5 minutes and night-time extension splinting in a custom-made plastic splint (Fig. 3)
- Full-time playing as soon as possible (usually at 2½–4 weeks), although performance is usually delayed for 6–8 weeks. Use of night-time splint in extension for additional 6–8 weeks
- Use of additional daytime abducting splints if needed from 1 to 6 weeks where wide span is required
- If skin grafts have been used, the initial period of absolute rest, compression dressing and splintage is prolonged for an additional 7 days.

digital contracture. Conversely, with many string players where the hand is held in the flexed position while playing, even significant digital contracture may not cause any technical

Results

Using the principles and techniques outlined for release of Dupuytren's contractures over the last 11 years in professional musicians (see Table 1) we have been able to avoid the disasters of digital nerve injury and haematoma and have been able to achieve early wound healing facilitating a very early return to limited playing and a 100% success rate in return to performance in a small series of professional musicians. The results are similar in recreational musicians. Even in recurrent disease, excellent release has been achieved and the disease stabilized using a combination of 'Z'-plasty flaps and interpositional graft, and on two occasions professional musicians have been able to return to performing, when indeed they had been advised, much to their dismay, to give up their careers.

References

Elliott D (1988) The early history of contracture of the palmar fascia. *J Hand Surg* **14b**:246–53.

Gonzalez RI (1974) Open fasciotomy in full thickness skin graft in the correction of digital flexion deformity. In: Hueston JT, Tubiana R, eds. *Dupuytren's Disease*. Churchill Livingstone: Edinburgh: 123–7.

Hueston JT (1961) Limited fasciectomy. *Plast Reconstr Surg* **27**:569–85.

Hueston JT (1984) The unfavourable results in Dupuytren's Disease. In: Goldwyn R, ed. *The Unfavourable Results in Plastic Surgery*, vol. 2. Little, Brown: Boston: 1031–41.

Logan AM, Brown HG, Louis-Smith B (1985) Radical digital dermofasciectomy in Dupuytren's Disease. *J Hand Surg* **10b**:353–7.

McCash CR (1964) The open palm technique in Dupuytren's contracture. *Br J Plast Surg* **17**:271–80.

Winspur I (1980) Dupuytren's contracture. In: Eisman B, ed. *Prognosis of Surgical Disease*. Saunders: Philadelphia: 500–501.

9
Nerve compression syndromes

Ian Winspur

When one considers the tortuous course of peripheral nerves in humans from the intervertebral foramina to the fingertips it is amazing that more do not suffer from significant nerve compressions at multiple sites. Indeed, considering that musicians spend so much of their time in fixed abnormal positions, their necks twisted and elbows bent, it is amazing that these conditions are not seen more commonly in this group of people. The incidence of true nerve entrapment in musicians seems to be very similar, if not slightly below, that in the general public (Lederman 1994). However, the differing presentation of these conditions in musicians and the possibility of confusion with related conditions and the specific modifications in analysis and treatment required for them all justify a separate chapter on nerve compression syndromes, even though the conditions are relatively uncommon.

Incidence

The true incidence of nerve compression syndromes (NCSs) among musicians is difficult to establish as the diagnoses from the various clinics tend to reflect the primary interest and specialty focus of that particular clinic. Hence in a series from London (Table 1) (Winspur and Wynn Parry 1997) NCS was diagnosed in 4% of all musicians presenting with upper arm complaints and this represented a 10% incidence among those diagnosed as having a recognized musculoskeletal disorder. Lederman (Lederman 1994) in his experience at the Cleveland Clinic found an incidence of 22.5% of NCS among all musicians presenting at this clinic, which represented 35% of those with a specific musculoskeletal diagnosis. Figures from the Mayo Clinic (Amadio and Russotti 1990) demonstrate a 22.5% incidence of

Table 1 Specific orthopaedic/rheumatological diagnoses in 323 patients attending Musicians' Clinic

True tenosynovitis	31
Rotator cuff/frozen shoulder	25
Old injury	17
Back strain	16
Osteoarthritis	11
Thoracic outlet	9
Tennis elbow	6
Ganglions	4
Carpal tunnel syndrome	4
Rheumatoid arthritis	3
Miscellaneous	11
	137 (42% of total)

NCS in patients diagnosed with a specific upper extremity musculoskeletal condition. Among these series of patients diagnosed with NCS there is a wide variation in the incidence of specific entrapment. However, by far and away the commonest conditions are carpal tunnel syndrome (CTS) and thoracic outlet syndrome (TOS); in the Mayo series CTS represents 57% of cases and TOS 26%; in the Cleveland series TOS represented 26% and CTS 21%; in the London series TOS 75% and CTS 25%. From these figures, however, it is obvious that NCSs constitute a significant cause of upper arm complaints in musicians and within this group of conditions the commonest specific syndromes are CTS and TOS. Ulnar nerve compression at the elbow, cubital tunnel syndrome (CubTS), was relatively common in the Cleveland series, but uncommon in the other two.

Anatomy of compression

Running from the neck distally, the nerves of the upper extremity run through several tight spaces. At each of these spaces the nerve can be compressed by external structures, or swelling and tumour. The actual mechanism of compression can be static – a rigid tunnel such as carpal tunnel, Guyon's canal or intervertebral foramen – or dynamic – the muscle bellies of pronator teres or supinator. Compression may also be exerted by the tight fascial edges of muscles – the proximal fibrous edge of the sublimis, supinator and scalene muscles. These tight spaces may also be constricted and narrowed by the coexistence of tumour or swelling in that space from non-nerve related structures, e.g. swelling of the tenosynovium in the carpal tunnel. The space may also be compressed through postural factors (TOS) or by prolonged non-physiological positioning of a joint (CTS and CubTS). Nerves at certain points must also glide around fixed bony prominences or in fixed canals. Nerve gliding is now recognized as an important physical attribute of a peripheral nerve. The ulnar nerve has been shown to glide 5–7 mm around a fixed bony point on the medial epicondyle of the elbow with elbow flexion and the median nerve has been demonstrated to glide between 7 mm and 14 mm in the carpal tunnel during wrist movement (Wilgis and Murphy 1986). When gliding is restricted either by external compression on the nerve or directly by tethering or scarring of the nerve, then indeed stretching injuries and microinjury occur to the nerve resulting in similar symptoms and signs to nerve compression. However, whether this small amount of gliding demonstrated in the peripheral nerves over fixed bony points, and the apparent clinical correlation of the loss of gliding to symptomatology, is sufficient scientific proof to support the hypothesis of 'adverse neural tension' in the more proximal nerves is questionable. Nevertheless physiotherapeutic regimes based on this hypothesis do seem to have some clinical benefit, perhaps related more to tightness of soft tissue structures consequent on prolonged abnormal postures.

small arteries and veins running in the loose mobile areolar tissue surrounding the nerve, tissue which also allows nerve gliding. This vascular supply then forms a precise external and internal network in and around the nerve, the maintenance of which is essential for the metabolic function of the nerve and the maintenance of correct interstitial pressure for important ion movement across the 'nerve–blood' barrier. This arrangement is highly susceptible to even small changes in pressure. The nerve itself is surrounded by a tough outer layer of epineurium which gives the nerve resistance to modest traction and external non-segmental pressure. The internal functioning of the axons, the active elements of the nerve, requires not only energy and ionic transfer, but also the physical transport of metabolites and active chemicals distally and proximally. These are carried via microtubular systems which themselves are affected by changes in pressure. Hence external pressure, particularly over a short segment, has multiple microanatomical effects on the peripheral nerve. These effects depend not only on the location of the pressure, but also on the duration and magnitude of the pressure. Small transitory changes will alter function and conductivity without causing physical damage to the nerve. Greater compression, particularly over longer periods and of greater force, will result in physical damage to the nerve both externally, fibrosing the epineurium and causing physical narrowing of the nerve at that point, and more importantly causing development of scar internally. The specific symptoms produced, particularly their pattern and cycle of development and recovery, relate directly to the duration and magnitude of compression. The long-term recoverability also relates to the extent of physical damage. The detection of abnormal nerve conduction when only transitory defects exist is not possible clinically. But this is a useful tool in many circumstances to confirm conduction abnormalities associated with continued compression and some degree of nerve damage.

Pathophysiology

Nerves are living structures not conduits (Lundborg and Danlin 1992). The blood supply to a peripheral nerve is provided by a network of

Double crush

Many of the common entrapment neuropathies were originally described in the nineteenth century. However, it is only in the last 50 years that clinicians have become fully alert to nerve compression as a source of pain as well as neurological defect. Clinicians have also become aware of an increase in distal nerve entrapment (CTS and CubTS) in patients with known proximal nerve compression either in the cervical spine or root of the neck (Mackinnon 1992). Upton (Upton and McComas 1973) proposed the hypothesis of 'double crush'. This term has now been modified to 'double-lesion neuropathy'. The hypothesis attempts to explain the significance of subclinical compression at two levels and it certainly fits with current knowledge of antegrade and retrograde axonal flow. The hypothesis has been proved experimentally in animals by double banding of peripheral nerves to subinjurious levels. The hypothesis may also be part of the explanation for the clinical observations that carpal tunnel syndrome is more frequent in patients with diabetes. One commonly observed phenomenon in patients with symptoms of both proximal and distal pressure, e.g. cervical spondylosis and CTS, is that relief of one component often relieves symptoms of the other. There may be a minimal level of neural activity at spinal level that needs to be exceeded for symptoms. If there are two levels of nociception, they summate. The role of dynamic multiple level nerve compression has also been postulated as a cause of 'industrial arm pain'. This is fascinating but unproven. However, it may be of some significance when dealing with musicians with arm pain, particularly related to poor posture, poor technique and muscle tension from extremely prolonged playing.

Diagnosis of compression neuropathy

The cardinal signs in diagnosing compression of a peripheral nerve are the development of sensory or motor disturbances distally in the specific distribution of the nerve in question (Lister 1993). However, many nerve compressions in their early stages produce only pain. It is also possible to develop the symptoms of dysaesthesia and paraesthesia in the apparent distribution of a particular peripheral nerve without that nerve being compressed – it can be related to adjacent tendon or tenosynovial swelling or oedema or more proximal non-compressive causes. With increased awareness of distal compression neuropathies, it is very easy and tempting to label any distal sensory upset as one of the known nerve compression syndromes. This occurs with unfortunate frequency and in dealing with the musician's arm, this leads to incomplete analysis of the true condition and its relationship to the instrument and playing, and to inappropriate and sometimes damaging treatment. Therefore the diagnosis of a specific entrapment syndrome should be made only when strict diagnostic, and in some situations, electrodiagnostic, criteria have been met.

Electrodiagnostic testing

Neurophysiological testing is an important adjunct to clinical diagnosis in NCS. Electromyography (EMG) using needle electrodes and calculation of nerve conduction velocity and delay (NCT) are both utilized (Wynn Parry 1981). Testing is entirely related to the skill of the tester and the tester should be clinically attuned and should be prepared to make non-standard comparison studies in every clinical situation. Musicians generally resist testing, being reluctant to have needles inserted into or electrical shocks given to areas upon which they rely for their livelihood. However, when the importance of the test and the reasons for testing are explained, they will usually submit. NCT is the most valuable test in localizing the specific area of segmental injury or compression and it is particularly valuable in the confirmation of CTS and CubTS. Both motor and sensory testing are utilized. Although a normal result cannot rule out early or intermittent compression, a negative result in CTS and CubTS in musicians should serve as a contraindication to surgical release. Neither NCT nor EMG have proved to be of great value diagnostically in TOS and are of no value in radial tunnel syndrome (RTS). However, it can be of value in the diagnosis and evaluation of possible double crush phenomenon and also in the exclusion of generalized peripheral neuropathies. There are, however, pitfalls: dynamic compression will not show; NCT only measures conductivity in large myelinated fibres and these constitute only a small portion of the nerve; anatomical variations exist; nerve conduction velocity falls off with age. Therefore, provided the deficiencies and pitfalls of testing are appreciated and the tester is clinically skilled, these tests can be of great value although not being necessarily diagnostic. When dealing with CTS and CubTS in musicians, the absence of slowing on NCT should be considered a contraindication to surgical decompression.

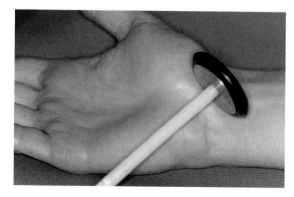

Figure 1

Tinel's sign being elicited over the median nerve at the wrist. In patients with cubital tunnel syndrome and carpal tunnel syndrome a positive test will commonly be present at the site of compression.

Nerve compression syndromes – general clinical presentation

CTS was first described in 1854 by Paget and CubTS (by another name) by Ramsey Hunt in 1908. In all these early cases the diagnosis was based on profound distal motor and sensory loss in the distribution of the involved nerve. To allow the condition to deteriorate to such a severe degree is unacceptable in modern times. Indeed in musicians, even the smallest degree of functional loss may be incompatible with playing and therefore musicians will present when only the very earliest of symptoms are present and before clear neurological changes have developed. In this situation, diagnosing is a much more demanding task. It is recognized that the earliest symptom of nerve compression is probably pain and aching. This is typically but not necessarily nocturnal, will awaken the patient from sleep and may be accompanied by paraesthesia in the sensory distribution of the nerve. However, if the nerve involved is purely motor, no paraesthesia may be present and the only symptom may be pain existing long before compression is sustained or severe enough to cause motor loss. The pain of nerve compression may be at the point of compression, but more commonly proximal to the site of compression, e.g. upper arm and shoulder aching in patients with CTS. The proximal referral of pain occurs not only when a predominantly sensory nerve is involved, but also when a purely motor nerve is involved. This is due to the fact that a 'pure' motor nerve also carries afferent fibres from joints and muscles.

The second important general sign for compression of a peripheral nerve is local tenderness on the nerve at the site of compression and the presence of Tinel's sign, the classical test (Fig. 1). When the nerve is percussed at the site of compression, paraesthesias are produced at that site and also sometimes distally. It is unusual not to have such signs present when significant nerve compression exists. Hence patients with TOS usually have deep tenderness in the supraclavicular area or at the base of the neck, patients with RTS have deep tenderness over the radial nerve within the extensor muscle mass in the proximal forearm and patients with CubTS have a positive Tinel's sign on palpating or percussing the ulnar nerve at the elbow. When such signs are not present, one has to be guarded in making the diagnosis of nerve compression.

The pain or paraesthesias produced by nerve compression can often be reproduced by provocative testing. When compression is induced by posture, extreme positioning of the involved joint (cf. extreme elbow flexion for CubTS or extreme wrist flexion for CTS) should produce symptoms. When a dynamic source is expected, resisted action of the involved muscle or muscles should reproduce symptoms (extensor carpi radialis brevis, ECRB, in RTS). Of course if there are other injured structures in the vicinity of the nerve, or suspected site of nerve compression, one has to ensure that these are not causing the patient's symptoms rather than the nerve pathology.

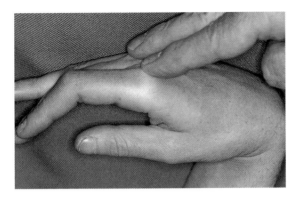

Figure 2

Phalen's test. Forced flexion of the wrist should be painless but produce paraesthesia in under 60 seconds. In patients with tenosynovitis of the flexor tendons at the wrist the manoeuvre is immediately uncomfortable.

Carpal tunnel syndrome in musicians

CTS is the commonest compression neuropathy seen both in the general population and in musicians. It is also the commonest misdiagnosis and incorrect label applied to musicians with arm and hand pain, tingling and numbness. It is therefore worth considering the condition in some detail. CTS refers to compression of the median nerve at the wrist as it lies within the carpal tunnel producing a specific set of symptoms and signs (Tubiana and Brockman 1991). The compression may occur because the rigid tunnel formed by the carpal bones and roofed by the strong rigid transverse carpal ligament is too tight, or because the volume of tissue within the tunnel is too great. The median nerve lying directly under the flexor retinaculum is subject to compression by the ligament – many times at its proximal and distal edges – and symptoms and signs of median nerve compression develop. It has been shown, however, that when the wrist is hyperflexed, the volume of the canal is reduced and the nerve can be physically compressed (Gelberman et al 1981). This is an important phenomenon when dealing with musicians, particularly guitarists. It is also the basis of the diagnostic provocative test (Phalen's test) (Fig. 2) and is one of the reasons patients with CTS develop symptoms at night while sleeping in the foetal position.

True sensory and motor disturbances are late signs in NCS. In a musician, falling performance will have precipitated cries for help long before these signs are present. However, transitory sensory disturbances may be seen early on and these need to be mapped out carefully and must be shown to lie within the discrete area of sensory distribution of that nerve for a diagnosis of isolated nerve compression to be made. This sensory mapping can be performed quickly using only the modalities of light touch or pinprick, although for more accurate recording, two-point discrimination and moving two-point discrimination must be used. The phenomenon exists also where the sensation is normal but the finger feels 'asleep'. This is called dysaesthesia and is frequently found in early sensory nerve compression. It is difficult to map. Motor disturbance is a late sign in NCS and the musician will have presented long before this is present. But subtle dysaesthesia and minimal motor loss may cause clumsiness in patients with CTS and indeed the presentation of CTS in musicians may simply be of nocturnal shoulder pain and slight clumsiness – not the symptoms one would normally expect from CTS. The treating physician must therefore be constantly on the alert for NCS as a cause for apparently bizarre symptoms in musicians.

Symptoms and signs

Compression of the median nerve at the wrist produces paraesthesias in the median distribution, nocturnal pain and aching in the upper arm and shoulder, sensory disturbance in the median distribution in the fingers (not including the palm which is supplied by a median nerve branch which does not pass through the carpal tunnel) and motor loss causing weakness and wasting of the thenar muscles. Sensory and motor loss are late signs and therefore are not commonly seen in musicians. Indeed the commonest presentation in musicians is of nocturnal dysaesthesia or slightly altered feeling in the fingers in association with nocturnal arm and shoulder aching.

The clinical signs of CTS are sensory alteration clearly limited to the distribution of the median nerve distally, thenar muscle wasting and loss of powerful thumb rotation, a positive Tinel's sign over the median nerve at the wrist and positive provocative testing with the wrist hyperflexed, producing paraesthesia and numbness within 60 seconds. At least two of the cardinal symptoms and two of the cardinal signs should be present before clinical diagnosis can be made. If nocturnal symptoms are not present then one should be very sceptical of the diagnosis.

Differential diagnosis

The differential diagnosis obviously includes all possible causes of median motor and sensory neuropathy, both proximally and distally. General and systemic causes of a peripheral polyneuropathy also have to be ruled out. More proximal compression of the median nerve either in the mid-forearm (pronator syndrome) or of the more proximal nerve trunks and nerve roots must also be excluded. Tumours and swellings within the carpal tunnel must also be ruled out and in this regard, when dealing with musicians, non-specific flexor tenosynovitis of the flexor tendons at the wrist and within the carpal tunnel is by far and away the most common cause of transient symptoms in the median distribution. This is specifically seen in violinists in the left hand and in keyboard players and pianists in both hands. In fact, in practical terms, the differential diagnosis of CTS in musicians falls into three subgroups:

- Classical idiopathic CTS
- Acute positional CTS
- Flexor tenosynovitis (FTS) of the wrist.

The principal differentiating features of these conditions are shown in Table 2.

In summary, the critical factors differentiating true median nerve compression at the wrist (CTS) from acute positional median nerve irritation and flexor tenosynovitis of the wrist without true compression are the presence of nocturnal symptoms and the presence of slowing of nerve conduction. Hence, in dealing with a musician in which the clinical diagnosis cannot be firmly made, nerve conduction testing is a necessary diagnostic step.

Acute positional CTS

This condition should be suspected in all guitarists presenting with symptoms of median nerve irritation at the wrist. However, the history will be subtly different in as much as the patient will complain of paraesthesia and numbness in the median distribution when playing and shortly after playing. He will not complain of symptoms when resting and he will not complain of nocturnal symptoms. The clinical examination will be entirely normal, apart from a positive Phalen's test and, when observing the guitarist playing, it will be noted how rotated he is holding the instrument and how hyperflexed his left wrist is held during playing (Fig. 3). Many guitarists are self-taught and this poor positioning of the instrument may be deliberate mimicking of a musical idol who also is mishandling the guitar. Also the wide-necked twelve-string guitar tends to encourage this malpositioning of the left wrist. The treatment of the condition in guitarists obviously requires modification of technique with possibly a change in instrument. This should be supervised by a suitable guitar

Table 2 Differential diagnosis of carpal tunnel syndrome

	Daytime symptoms	Nocturnal symptoms	Phalen's	Tinel's	Swelling	NCT
CTS	0	+	+	+	0	+
Acute positional	+	0	+	0	0	0
FTS	+	0	*	0	+	0

*Palen's manoeuvre (forced flexion of the wrist) produces marked discomfort in patients with FTS of the finger flexors at the wrist, which in itself is a useful clinical sign.

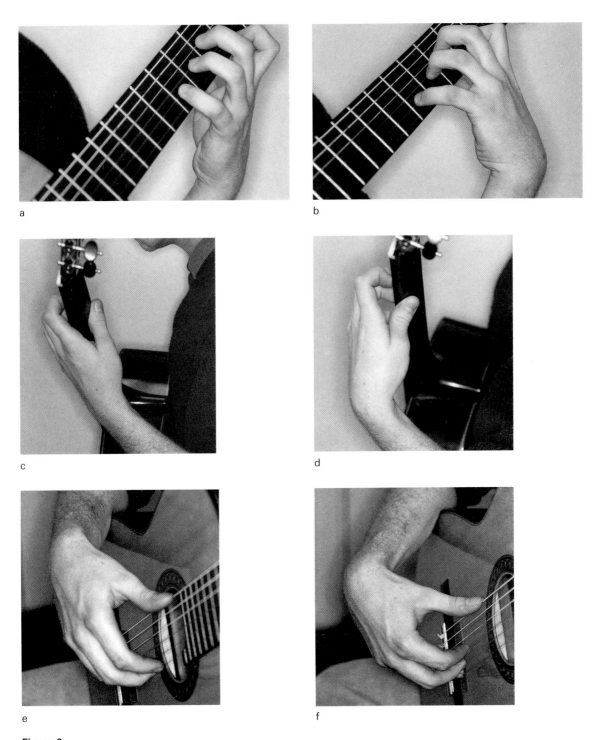

Figure 3

(a–f) Overrotation of the guitar, producing hyperflexion of the right wrist while playing, with a high risk of producing symptoms due to compression on the median nerve at the wrist.

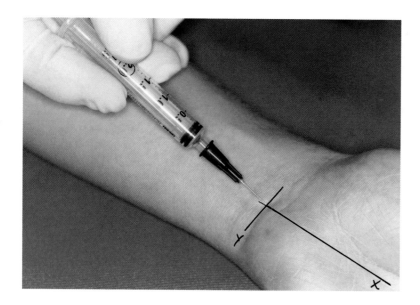

Figure 4

Injection of the carpal tunnel: this is the safe technique, avoiding any risk of direct injury to the median nerve. Note short needle. Axis Y = 1 cm proximal to wrist crease. Axis X = extension of mid-line of ring finger. If the needle is positioned too far ulnarward direct injury to the ulnar nerve may occur.

teacher. These patients fare badly following unnecessary surgical release.

Flexor tenosynovitis of the wrist

Keyboard players present complaining of numbness in the median innervated fingers, usually occurring while playing or shortly after playing. On careful questioning it usually emerges that these symptoms follow a period of intense practice, prolonged practice of unfamiliar difficult pieces or prolonged performance. The symptoms occur in either hand. When the symptoms are at their worst the patients may complain of occasional nocturnal symptoms, but nocturnal symptoms do not predominate. The symptoms are not present when the musician has a break from playing, while he is on holiday or limits his playing. Examination will show boggy swelling at the wrist also involving commonly the flexor tendons to the long finger, which will also be swollen, nodular and tender. There will be a lack of specific findings in relation to the median nerve at the wrist and Phalen's manoeuvre will produce discomfort but no paraesthesia. Nerve conduction tests will be normal. The patient has flexor tenosynovitis, a

transient swelling of the wrist tenosynovium which is causing temporary dysfunction in the adjacent median nerve from oedema rather than true sustained pressure. This same classical picture can be seen in violinists when playing complex pieces requiring excessive vibrato. The treatment for flexor tenosynovitis of the wrist is conservative and most certainly non-surgical, even if neurological symptoms seem to predominate. A reduction (not a cessation) in playing and critical analysis of technique and instrument – particularly the weight of the piano action – is obligatory. Oral anti-inflammatory medicine will help. Injection of non-absorbable steroid into the carpal canal, with careful avoidance of direct injury to the median nerve, can be of great value with rapid onset of action and relief of symptoms (Fig. 4). Surgery is not indicated unless NCT is abnormal and surgery even when indicated gives dismal results and should only be considered as a last resort.

Classical CTS

In musicians with early symptoms of the disease, relief of symptoms can many times be achieved using night splints or anti-inflammatory medicine and some modification in playing. Believers also swear of the benefits of large doses of oral B6 and acupuncture. However, when the condition is well established, and NCTs are positive, surgical decompression is usually required to provide permanent relief. The fact that the patient is a musician should be no contraindication. The standard surgical techniques should be used. Clear visualization of the median nerve is imperative, and therefore the open technique using a palmar incision is to be recommended in musicians rather than the endoscopic techniques, where there is slightly increased chance of serious nerve injury. The incisions should not cross the wrist crease unless formal exploration of the distal forearm is required. Postoperatively the wrist should be splinted in slight extension for a few days to minimize the chance of postoperative bowstringing or dislocation of the flexor tendons, a disaster in a musician. Gentle finger exercises and light playing for short periods is started immediately postoperative elevation ceases – usually at 36 hours. Removable wrist splintage with the wrist in slight extension is started at 5 days, when full practice can be resumed, but full sustained wrist flexion is not allowed till 10–12 days following surgery. The results of surgery can be expected to be as dramatically effective as those in the general population and this has been confirmed in published series in musicians (Lederman 1994). In our experience, all patients have returned to full playing rapidly with the exception of one who, while clearly suffering CTS as shown by positive NCT, also proved to have a double-crush lesion with C6, 7 and 8 radiculopathy also requiring surgical decompression. Indeed the commonest cause of failure following carpal tunnel release in musicians is incorrect diagnosis, once again confirming the importance of making a very accurate diagnosis and not labelling just any distal neuropathy as 'carpal tunnel syndrome'.

Ulnar nerve entrapment

Ulnar nerve entrapment most frequently occurs at the elbow (CubTS), where the ulnar nerve passes round the medial epicondyle and is stretched when the elbow is flexed, particularly if there is loss of nerve gliding due to local inflammation or compression from the fibrous arch of the origin of flexor carpi ulnaris or the fibrous rim of the medial intramuscular septum. It is estimated that approximately 15% of the general population demonstrate asymptomatic or transiently symptomatic ulnar nerve anterior dislocation with elbow flexion (Macnicol 1987). Given that so many musicians play with elbows flexed for long periods, it is surprising that ulnar nerve compression of the elbow is not more common. The ulnar nerve can also be compressed distally at the wrist or its deep motor branch in the hand. Compression at these other sites is usually related to prior fracture or local benign tumour and is rare in musicians, although it has been recorded in flautists (Brockman et al 1991).

CubTS presents classically as sensory loss in the ulnar distribution involving the little and half the ring fingers, insidious motor loss involving the intrinsic muscles of the hand which may only be detected by measurement of grip strength and also loss of power in the ulnar-supplied long flexors of the fingers (flexor digitorum profundus to the little and sometimes the ring). However, these signs are all late in developing and the early presentation usually seen in musicians is of aching around the elbow and dysaesthesia in the little and ring fingers. The dysaesthesia will commonly be worse at night related to elbow positioning. Indeed, when this is the only symptom and postural reasons can be identified and explained to the musician, provided he does not require elbow flexion for playing (non-string players) careful avoidance of prolonged elbow flexion during sleep, while driving or while on the telephone may be enough to eliminate all symptoms. The principal differential diagnosis when considering CubTS are C8–T1 radiculopathy and irritation of the lower trunks of the brachial plexus in one of the many conditions considered under the general title thoracic outlet syndrome (TOS).

When the ulnar nerve is irritated in the cubital tunnel, the nerve is usually tender and sensitive and a strongly positive Tinel's sign is usually present (Fig. 5). When this is not present one must be sceptical of the diagnosis. The diagnosis should be confirmed by NCT. Although normal NCT does not exclude early or transient compression, one should not consider surgical

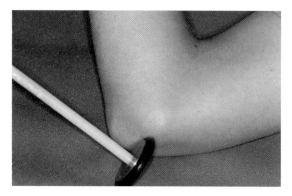

Figure 5

Eliciting Tinel's sign over the ulnar nerve in the cubital tunnel.

intervention on the ulnar nerve at the elbow in musicians unless NCTs are abnormal.

Treatment of the early cases should always be conservative. This means providing advice on sleeping and driving positions. It also means examining the patients and analysing while they play in the hope that their playing technique may be partly responsible and that with minor modification of technique or instrument, prolonged extreme elbow flexion can be avoided. If conservative measures fail or are inapplicable as in violinists, and if NCT is positive, one should consider surgical release if the patient's symptoms are sufficient and particularly if the patient's musical performance is failing. We know of three professional musicians (a pianist, a violinist and a viola player) who have had highly successful decompressions and Lederman described a 50% success rate in four cases. This raises the question of which operation – simple decompression versus decompression and transposition – and which method of transposition. There are advocates of simple decompression alone (by releasing the fibrous arch of flexor carpi ulnaris, FCU), but this is controversial and high recurrence rates have been recorded in some series. Additionally, when dealing with musicians who tend to spend long periods playing with their elbows flexed, it is logical to recommend transposition at the same time as

decompression to prevent the constant traction associated with prolonged elbow flexion.

The next question is which method of transposition – the simpler subcutaneous transposition with the lower morbidity, or submuscular transposition or epicondylectomy which are both associated with a considerably more prolonged postoperative morbidity and elbow stiffness and an increased risk of long-term elbow stiffness (Eversman 1993). There is no clear proven value of the more complicated methods, particularly in the primary cases, and therefore when dealing with musicians, when early return to limited playing is so critical, we believe strongly that the simpler, subcutaneous anterior transposition with lower morbidity is the procedure of choice. It must however be performed accurately with complete release of the nerve proximally and completed without the kinks and twists distally so often seen when surgical pulleys and tunnels are created. We personally use soft tissue closure of the cubital tunnel itself and the solid subcutaneous suture of the posterior flap as the method of securing tension-free, unkinked anterior location of the released ulnar nerve.

In summary, CubTS does occur in musicians, but not with the frequency one would expect. Most of these cases can be treated by conservative means and fare satisfactorily. However, when conservative measures have failed and the diagnosis is confirmed by NCT, surgical release can be performed in musicians with very satisfactory results. The nerve should be transposed at the time of decompression and we feel that the simpler subcutaneous placement of the nerve is the procedure of choice because of the shorter rehabilitation period and the much reduced chance of permanent elbow stiffness.

Radial nerve entrapment

Radial nerve entrapment is one of the more unusual compression neuropathies seen in the general population and similarly so in musicians. However, it is important for two reasons:

• It may be the cause of persisting and unresolving symptoms of tennis elbow type
• Patients with aching arms and tenderness associated with prolonged playing and

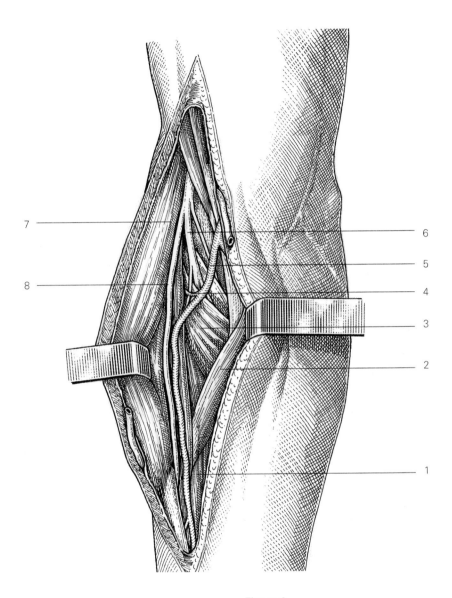

7

8

6

5

4

3

2

1

misuse often show transitory signs of irritation or compression of their radial nerves in
the proximal forearm.

The radial nerve passes from the upper arm into
the forearm in front of the elbow joint, then
radial to the radial head and from there posterior
to the proximal radius, and provides motor
branches to the extensor muscles via its main
trunk and a terminal motor branch, the posterior
interosseous nerve, and sensation over the
dorsum of the radial two-thirds of the hand via
its superficial sensory branch (see Fig. 6). The

Figure 6

Anatomy of radial nerve in the radial tunnel: 1, flexor carpi
radialis; 2, pronator teres; 3, supinator; 4, radial recurrent
artery; 5, radial artery; 6, posterior interosseous nerve;
7, brachioradialis; 8, superficial sensory branch of radial
nerve. From Tubiana et al (1990).

1 flexor carpi radialis
2 pronator teres
3 supinator
4 radial recurrent artery
5 radial artery
6 posterior interosseous nerve
7 brachioradialis
8 superficial sensory branch of radial nerve

nerve may be trapped at a number of sites. When this involves the pure sensory branch (Wartenburg's syndrome) distal sensation is disturbed. When it involves the distal motor branch (posterior interosseous syndrome) (Maffulli and Maffulli 1991) motor loss to the distal extensors occurs. However, these signs are seldom seen in musicians as they occur late and also because the nerve is most commonly compressed more proximally as it runs in a tight space, the radial tunnel (Lawrence et al 1995), deep to brachioradialis and ECRB, eventually disappearing through a fibrous arch in the supinator in the proximal forearm. Compression in this area may be static (a leash of vessels crossing the nerve proximal to supinator or the fibrous edge of supinator, the arcade of Frohse). However, more commonly the compression is dynamic associated with muscle swelling, oedema or indeed a more proximal injury as seen in tennis elbow. The compressed nerve is tender over its course and provocative testing resisting the action of the common extensor to the long finger or ECRB and supinator reproduces symptoms. However, these manoeuvres will also reproduce symptoms in tennis elbow. NCT is of little value as the nerve is deep to muscles and difficult to isolate, and since in many cases the compression is dynamic. However, musicians presenting with persisting dull proximal arm pain, tennis elbow type of pain or resistant tennis elbow should all be examined very carefully to exclude RTS. The diagnosis is based on a high index of suspicion, prompted by the patient's history and confirmed by persisting tenderness over the radial nerve (Fig. 7) in comparison to the non-affected nerve in the opposite forearm. This comparison is important because deep palpation of the radial nerve can be uncomfortable in normal arms and only increased discomfort is of diagnostic value.

The treatment of RTS is usually conservative – modified playing schedules, oral anti-inflammatory medicine, etc. Most will settle spontaneously and at least 6–9 months should be allowed before more aggressive treatment is considered in musicians. Unfortunately, one does not have the luxury of NCT as an indicator for surgical decompression. But if sufficient time has been allowed and the history and findings are consistent on multiple examinations then the nerve should be decompressed. This is done via

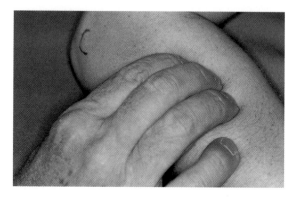

Figure 7

Testing for radial nerve tenderness (lateral epicondyle marked). Comparison with the non-involved side should always be made as the test can be uncomfortable even in normal arms.

a short transverse anterolateral incision 4–5 cm distal to the elbow flexion crease (Crawford 1984) and the nerve approached in the interval between brachioradialis and ECRB (Henry's Mobile Wad) and the forearm flexors. Splitting of brachioradial muscle belly is not necessary and increases postoperative pain. Complete release of the main trunk of the radial nerve and the superficial and deep branches from all fibrous brands and vascular arcades is mandatory, as is complete release of the arcade of Frohse and the myofascia of the supinator. Occasionally distal release of the supinator is also required.

The relief from the preoperative discomfort is usually dramatic and if not so one must question the diagnosis. Occasionally release of RTS is performed in conjunction with release of tennis elbow. Tennis elbow releases themselves in musicians are not reliable and if one is faced with releasing both the radial nerve and a tennis elbow in a musician, one must admit the musician's playing career may be in jeopardy.

Thoracic outlet syndrome (TOS)

TOS is a clinical term referring to a symptom/sign complex of conditions causing neurovascular disturbances in the root of the neck. Many

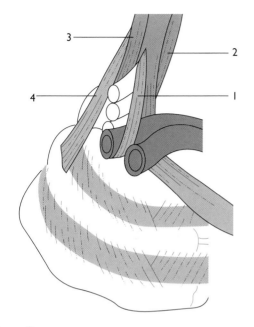

Figure 8

Thoracic outlet: the brachial plexus, subclavian vessels and scalene muscles at the level of the first rib. 1, Prescalene fibrous band; 2, anterior scalene; 3, middle scalene; 4, posterior scalene. From Narakas (1993).

structures have been implicated in causing compression. Classically these have included extra cervical ribs and bands which have been shown to distort the subclavian artery causing multiple emboli and thrombosis. The scalene muscles and first rib have also been incriminated, distorting the lower roots and trunks of the brachial plexus causing predominantly neurological disturbances. Often, however, no precise single structure can be implicated and the compression in many patients – and this is particularly true of musicians – is most probably dynamic due to the effects of abnormal positioning of the shoulder girdle and neck on the tight triangular space formed by the clavicle and scapula in relationship to the fixed bony thorax (see Fig. 8). The clinical presentation of TOS in musicians is described in Chapter 7. The diagnosis is basically clinical and most of the so-called provocative tests are not diagnostic. Similarly, electrodiagnostic testing may be useful in

excluding distal compression neuropathy from the differential diagnosis, but it is of no value directly in confirming the diagnosis of TOS.

Generally, symptoms suggestive of TOS include neck pain, discomfort and aching in the root of the neck and arm, particularly when working with arms raised or elevated; nocturnal aching in the shoulder and arm; inner arm and elbow pain and paraesthesia in the hand, particularly in the ring and little fingers. In this regard, it must be differentiated from ulnar nerve compression symptoms which differ in their pain distribution and the area of sensory loss in the inner arm and elbow. As with other compression neuropathies, the signs of sensory loss and motor loss are late and are not usually present in musicians. The area of referral of pain and of dysaesthesia is usually the inner aspects of the elbow and proximal forearm and this distinguishes TOS from CubTS. Subtle motor loss may be present and may involve both the intrinsic muscles of the hand and the extrinsic flexors. NCT will be helpful in differentiating CubTS from TOS but is not diagnostically accurate enough to make a firm diagnosis of TOS. The signs of subclavian compromise (Adson's test) when the radial pulse is diminished by high elevation of the hand and rotation of the neck are not reliable. MRI scanning of the root of the neck with modern high resolution equipment and MRI angiography (without the need for intra-arterial injection – a technique usually resisted by the musician patient) can sometimes be diagnostic when static compression exists. The diagnosis, however, is generally made on clinical grounds, appropriate symptoms in association with compatible clinical findings distally and, often, discomfort to deep palpation in the root of the neck.

The diagnosis of TOS is one of the commonest made in musicians' clinics in patients suffering from nerve compression syndromes. This may relate to the non-specific nature of the condition, the protean manifestations of TOS or that indeed musicians commonly suffer dynamic compression in the root of the neck because of the unique physical demands made on them when playing. Much has been made of the surgical treatment of TOS and indeed of the successful surgical treatment of TOS in musicians. But other experienced clinicians have drawn attention to the dangers associated with these operations (Leffert 1991) and also to the fact that most

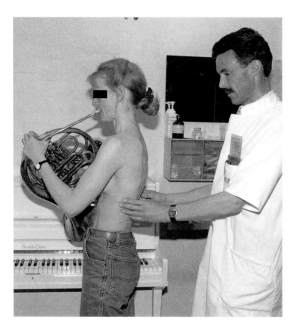

Figure 9

Examination of the patient's neck, shoulder and thoracic spine while the patient is playing (by courtesy of Dr ABM Rietveld).

patient will be different and a specific exercise beneficial for one may dramatically aggravate the condition or produce new symptoms in another, and should be abandoned. These patients may also be suffering sleep disruption and reactive depression, both of which need to be addressed.

In summary, TOS is a common diagnosis in musicians with upper extremity musculoskeletal disorders. It is a clinical diagnosis and is often used imprecisely. Electrodiagnostic testing is not of value apart from the exclusion of distal compression neuropathies. The treatment for most cases is conservative and most will respond well. Surgery should only be considered for those with severe symptoms in whom conservative measures have completely failed and the patient should be warned of the risks from this major operation. Nevertheless, there are documented cases of musicians having satisfactorily returned to playing after release of the TOS, usually by first rib resection.

musicians will improve without surgery. Indeed, in a series from the musicians' clinic in London, where 9 patients were diagnosed as having TOS out of 132 with 'organic conditions of the upper extremity', all TOS cases were treated conservatively and all recovered completely. Whether this indicates that the term TOS is used imprecisely or that indeed the patient with true static compression due to abnormal structures is very rare, is difficult to assess.

The non-surgical care of musicians with TOS consists of a careful analysis of the arm and neck position which produces the musician's symptoms while playing (Fig. 9). This must be assessed while the musician is actually playing. Treatment should be supportive with simple analgesics and NSAIDs may also help. Physical therapy to improve neck and body positioning and upper body stamina is the sheet anchor of treatment. This needs to be performed by a skilled and sympathetic physiotherapist, for each

Digital nerve compression

The commonest digital nerve compression syndrome is called 'bowler's thumb'. In this condition constant irritating pressure over the ulnar digital nerve of the right hand of ten pin bowlers when holding the bowling ball causes steady development of a painful neuroma on that nerve with distal sensory disturbance. A similar lesion has been seen on the thumbs of French horn players. If the patient stops bowling the neuroma resolves. If that is not practical steroid injections around the involved nerve are beneficial. Similar neuromas have been described in violinists, harpists, guitarists and in the left index finger of flautists. If one observes how many professional cellists practise and play with self-adhesive dressings on their fingertips, the suspicion is raised that small distal digital neuromas are more common than acknowledged. A very unusual but recorded pulp neuroma in a violinist (Dobyns 1992) was shown to be a pacinian corpuscle tumour, a hyperplasia of one of the types of nerve end organs. This lesion will not settle spontaneously and can only be treated by surgical removal, which may leave a small area of sensory loss on the pulp. This may be of considerable detriment to the musician and consideration needs to be given therefore before surgery is performed in this type of situation.

Conclusion

In summary, NCSs do occur in musicians but not with the frequency one would expect. The presentation in musicians is earlier and before the classical signs of sensory and motor loss have developed. The commonest presentation is pain and indeed NCSs should always be considered when assessing a musician with a painful arm. However the diagnosis of a specific NCS should only be made when strict clinical criteria are met and in most circumstances when confirmed by NCT. Most cases can be treated conservatively but a small number will require surgical release. The indications for surgery should be strict, but if the diagnosis is correct and the surgery performed with skill, the results, particularly in patients with CTS, should be as satisfactory as those in the general population.

References

Amadio PC, Russotti G (1990) Evaluation and treatment of hand and wrist disorders in musicians. *Hand Clin* **6**:405–16.

Brockman R, Chamagne P, Tubiana R (1991) The upper extremity in musicians. In: Tubiana R, ed. *The Hand*, vol. 4. WB Saunders: Philadelphia: 873–85.

Crawford GP (1984) Radial tunnel syndrome. *J Hand Surg* **914**:451–2.

Dobyns J (1992) Digital nerve compression. *Hand Clin* **8**:359–67.

Eversman W (1993) Entrapment and compression neuropathies. In: Green D, ed. *Operative Hand Surgery*, vol. 2 (3rd edn). Churchill Livingstone: New York: 1356–65.

Gelberman R, Hergenroeder PT, Hargens AR et al (1981) The carpal tunnel syndrome. A study of carpal tunnel pressures. *J Bone Joint Surg* **63A**:680–3.

Lawrence Mobbs P, Fortems Y et al (1995) Radial tunnel syndrome. *J Hand Surg* **20B**:454–9.

Lederman R (1994) Neuromuscular problems in the performing arts. *Muscle Nerve* **17**:569–77.

Leffert RD (1991) Thoracic outlet syndrome. In: Tubiana R, ed. *The Hand*, vol. 4. WB Saunders: Philadelphia: 343–51.

Lister G (1993) Compression. In: Lister G, ed. *The Hand Diagnosis and Indications* (3rd edn). Churchill Livingstone: Edinburgh: 283–322.

Lundborg G, Dahlin L (1992) The pathophysiology of nerve compression. *Hand Clin* **8**:215–27.

Mackinnon SE (1992) Double and multiple crush syndromes. *Hand Clin* **8**:369–95.

Macnicol MF (1987) Entrapment neuropathies. In: Lamb D, ed. *The paralysed hand*. Churchill Livingstone: Edinburgh: 169–88.

Maffulli N, Maffulli F (1991) Transient entrapment neuropathy of the posterior interosseous nerve in violin players. *J Neurol Neurosurg Psychiatry* **54**:65–7.

Narakas A (1993) Cervico-brachial compression In: Tubiana R, ed. *The Hand*, vol. 4. WB Saunders: Philadelphia: 352–89.

Tubiana R, Brockman R (1991) General considerations in carpal tunnel syndrome. In: Tubiana R, ed. *The Hand*, vol. 4. WB Saunders: Philadelphia: 441–9.

Tubiana R, McCullough CJ, Masquelet AC (1990) *An Atlas of Surgical Exposures of the Upper Extremity*. Martin Dunitz: London.

Wilgis S, Murphy R (1986) The significance of longitudinal excursion in peripheral nerves. *Hand Clin* **2**:761–8.

Winspur I, Wynn Parry CB (1997) The musician's hand. *J Hand Surg* **22B**:433–40.

Wynn Parry C (1981) Electrodiagnosis. In: Wynn Parry C. *Rehabilitation of the Hand* (4th edn). Butterworth: London: 208–33.

10

Surgical management of trauma in musicians: going the extra mile

Ian Winspur

As far as severe injury is concerned, playing a musical instrument is a low-risk occupation. However, musicians drive cars. They also show a penchant for cooking and DIY (home improvements), and domestic accidents with sharp knives, electrical appliances and power tools occur with unfortunate frequency. Indeed, 20–30% of all operations performed on musicians result from these types of accident. Our own experience shows that of 34 operations performed over a 12-year period on professional musicians, 7 were for trauma:

- A completely amputated fingertip from a kitchen knife
- A completely divided double flexor tendon injury in a digit from a kitchen knife
- An extensive forearm laceration dividing muscles and partially dividing the median nerve in a fall through a glass kitchen door
- A severe fracture dislocation of a proximal interphalangeal (PIP) joint from softball
- An extensor tendon laceration from DIY
- A closed acute mallet deformity from bed-making
- A Bennett's fracture from brawling.

Musicians, despite the known risks to hand and fingers, do indulge in contact sports and the more dangerous ball games. Indeed, amazingly, a certain renowned English orchestra was involved recently in a charity cricket match – a sport notorious for finger injuries – and volunteered 11 of its finest from the woodwind and string sections. Fortunately no one was injured!

These types of injuries can have a devastating effect on the musicians involved. The general rule of thumb when dealing with such an injury to a musician's hand should be

'stable, anatomical repair' even if relative contraindications exist, and, if in doubt, extra effort should be made to achieve these goals in this group of patients.

Initially, the wound or closed injury should be assessed accurately and independently as in any patient. But when dealing with a musician, the impact of the injury on the functional needs of the musician should also be carefully analysed from the onset. The subsequent repair, reconstruction and any anticipated compromise are adjusted to meet the musician's needs. For example, an oblique amputation of a fingertip in a pianist, preserving the radial half of the pulp, should be treated initially by skin-grafting of the defect rather than by either bone-shortening or readjustment of intact sensate radial skin to cover an ulnar defect. This may seem obvious but small and devastating errors can be made if a full complete assessment of the musician's needs and his instrument is not made initially. Similarly, a clear rehabilitation plan should be made from the outset. Inappropriate and protracted immobilization can cause damaging stiffness, while lack of appropriate immobilization may cause displacement of fractures or rupture of incompletely lacerated or partially injured structures.

Open lacerations

A very accurate initial assessment of function in associated or potentially injured structures must be made (Fig. 1). If the integrity of any such structure cannot be clearly ascertained at the initial examination, then under optimum conditions

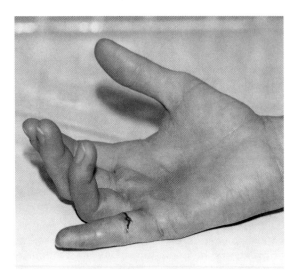

Figure 1

Laceration to flexor aspect of finger with little doubt about the injured structures (both flexor tendons and ulnar digital nerve). In less obvious cases, formal exploration may be a necessary early step to diagnosis and correct treatment in musicians.

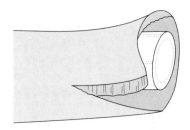

a

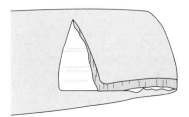

b

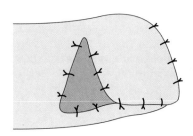

c

Figure 2

(a,b,c) Closure of fingertip amputation formally, without bone shortening, using a neurovascular flap created from the existing traumatic avulsion flap and small skin graft (redrawn from Winspur I 1983, with permission).

formal exploration of the wound should be performed. Accurate evaluation of all injured structures can then be made, formal repair performed as required and appropriate post-operative planning made. Fingertip amputation should be treated formally (Fig. 2) either by skin graft or appropriate local flap (Winspur 1983). In general, bone-shortening techniques should be avoided and existing undamaged tissue should only be utilized after full analysis of the musician's specific needs. The open techniques of fingertip treatment should be avoided because of the prolonged healing time.

Tendon lacerations

Partial tendon injuries, either flexor or extensor, if unrecognized can progress to complete rupture. However, if they are immobilized excessively adherence and stiffness will ensue. Partial flexor tendon injuries, if over 40–50% of the tendon is involved, may result in triggering. Therefore formal exploration, repair and appropriate postoperative care are mandatory if a significant flexor tendon injury is suspected. Complete tendon lacerations, flexor or extensor, have to be repaired as a primary procedure in the conventional way and postoperative mobilization techniques have to be used to maximize tendon gliding. If a profundus tendon is completely lacerated in isolation in zone 1 or 2, even through the sublimis tendon is intact,

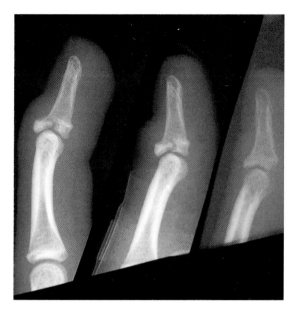

Figure 3

Treatment of mallet finger by splintage. The radiograph illustrates how, even with a sizeable fracture fragment, hyperextension reduces the fracture and if maintained for 6 weeks allows the extensor mechanism to reconstitute (by courtesy of Dr G Crawford).

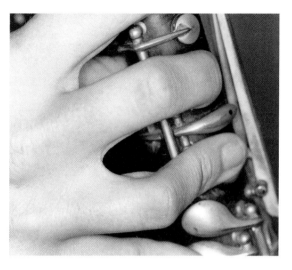

Figure 4

'Physiological' boutonnière positioning of the right ring finger on a 30-year-old female clarinet player.

formal repair (Leddy 1993) and protected early mobilization should always be performed in a musician. Excellent co-operation and compliance can be expected from the musician patient in the postoperative therapy period following this type of complex repair and the loss of existing active flexion at the PIP joint is unlikely to occur.

Closed tendon injuries

Two common closed injuries occur, the mallet deformity with or without avulsion fracture, and the closed boutonnière deformity. The mallet deformity follows a direct blow and may be complete or incomplete. In either circumstance it must be treated, although the period of absolute immobilization can be reduced for the incomplete lesion. The results of open and closed treatment and the periods of immobilization are very

similar (Crawford 1984) and therefore closed splintage by moulded plastic splint (Fig. 3) is the treatment of choice for the musician. Failure of closed treatment should be treated by operative repair and temporary k-wire fixation.

The boutonnière deformity can follow direct injury or can occur slowly by attrition in any condition where there is swelling around the dorsum of the PIP joint. The condition can be complete or incomplete (Zancolli 1979). Acute complete deformities in musicians should be formally repaired as this gives more predictable results with shortened immobilization times. Incomplete or subacute lesions should be treated by splintage in the standard fashion. Any injury causing swelling around the PIP joint in the musician should be treated by a short period of splinting of the PIP in full extension to prevent the development of the boutonnière deformity. In all cases where the PIP joint is splinted, the dorsal interphalangeal (DIP) joint must be left

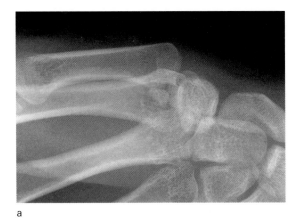
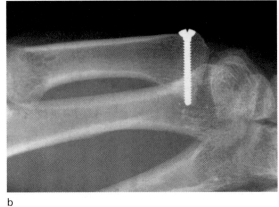

a   b

Figure 5

(a) Bennett's fracture. In this instance the volar fragment is small, but the metacarpal is nevertheless unstable with the carpometacarpal joint subluxing dorsally. (b) Stable anatomical reduction, allowing very early mobilization, is achieved by single compression screw fixation.

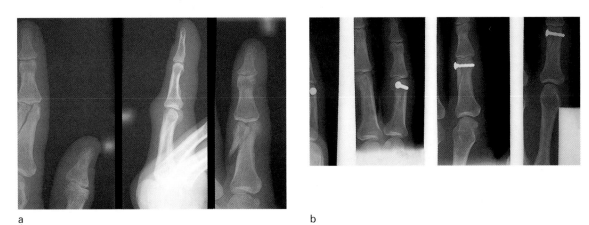

a   b

Figure 6

(a) Unstable intra-articular fracture. (b) Anatomically reduced and held physiologically with one compression screw allowing early range of motion (by courtesy of Dr G Crawford).

free and must be actively mobilized (see Chapter 11). This is of particular importance in musicians requiring hyperflexion of the distal joint (e.g. viola, cello). Occasionally, particularly in woodwind players, overenthusiastic correction of a pathological boutonnière deformity has to be tempered by the realization that the patient's playing position requires 'physiological' boutonnière positioning (Fig. 4).

Closed fractures

Fractures, in general, will be treated in the conventional way. However, there must be emphasis placed on the restoration of anatomical normality in involved joints and on early mobilization. This may lead to an earlier use of internal fixation than in the non-musician patient. Nowhere is this seen more clearly than in the

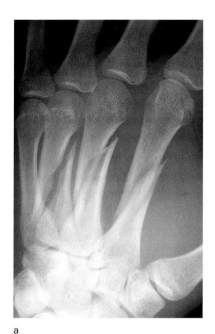
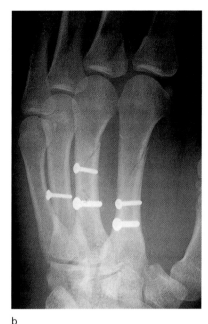

a   b

Figure 7

(a) Multiple rotated metacarpal fractures. (b) Open reduction correcting a functionally unacceptable deformity and allowing early mobilization (by courtesy of Dr G Crawford).

management of the Bennett fracture in the musician's thumb. All instrumentalists use both thumbs with the exception of the left thumb in trumpet players (and even this thumb is used continuously to turn the pages of music or to wipe the sweating brow). The Bennett's fracture, even if only slightly displaced, is a potentially unstable intra-articular fracture and the conflicting needs for an accurately reduced and maintained joint surface and early mobilization can only be achieved by very accurate stable early open reduction. The preferred approach is using a single compression screw which allows mobilization within 2–3 days of surgical reduction (Fig. 5). In phalangeal and metacarpal fractures no compromise should be accepted; intra-articular fractures should be anatomically reduced (Fig. 6); unstable rotated metacarpal and phalangeal fractures should also be openly reduced and fixed (Fig. 7) (Crawford 1976). Similarly, in closed wrist fractures, if satisfactory stable reduction and restoration of length, volar tilt, radiocarpal and distal radioulnar articulations cannot be achieved and maintained by closed

means, open reduction should be utilized at an early stage (Amadio 1995) (Fig. 8). Multiple complex injuries should be anatomically repaired if technically possible or otherwise reconstructed. Examples are given later in this chapter.

Nerve injuries

Laceration to a major peripheral nerve is a devastating injury for a musician. Indeed, even a partial laceration to a less important distal sensory nerve can also have profound effects. An established neuroma in continuity is a troublesome and extremely difficult condition to treat following partial nerve injury in a musician's hand and is to be avoided at all costs. The optimum results from these injuries can only be obtained by early recognition of the injury and early tension-free microsurgical repair of the nerve involved (Wilgis and Brushart 1993). (The exact technique of repair is probably of lesser importance.) Therefore, it is important that early

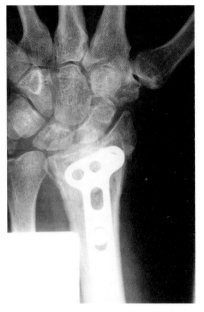

a

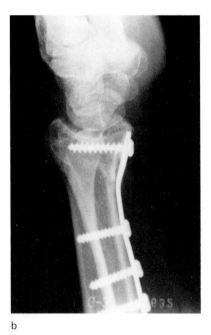

b

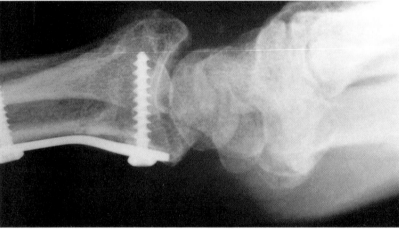

c

Figure 8

(a,b,c) A 60-year-old jazz saxo-phonist sustained a severe intra-articular fracture of his left wrist in a fall from his bicycle. Primary open reduc-tion was performed at his local orthopaedic hospital. The patient returned to limited playing 10 days after surgery and to full professional playing 8 weeks later. He presented 8 months after injury for plate removal because of recurrent swelling and flexor tenosyno-vitis of the wrist; he missed 1 week of playing following surgical removal of the plate.

accurate diagnosis of any nerve laceration be made, even, if necessary, by surgical exploration of a questionable injury and early accurate repair of the nerve achieved. This applies even to less important digital nerves distally and indeed any digital nerve injury in a musician should be repaired surgically up to and in some situations even beyond the DIP crease.

The following four cases are excellent examples of severe, potentially devastating injuries where early analysis of the musician's loss and needs and an aggressive approach by the surgeons involved has maximized the anatomical restora-tion. A less complex approach would not have provided the mechanical elements needed for these musicians to be able to continue playing.

Case report 1

Toe-to-hand transfer for thumb reconstruction in a professional bagpipe player

Stewart Watson

Patient

The patient was a 43-year-old male; this man was a professional bagpipe player and pipe major, keyboard player and guitarist.

He was admitted with a completely amputated left thumb, just distal to the metacarpophalangeal joint (Fig. 9a). The amputation was oblique through the base of the proximal phalanx comminuted into the metacarpophalangeal joint. The injury was sustained on a circular saw while doing DIY at home. An attempt at replantation was performed by an experienced consultant and senior registrar but it did not prove possible to arterialize the amputated part.

Circular saw injuries are by nature ragged, untidy injuries with a wide zone of injury and replantation is by no means certain in this type of injury but, of course, should be attempted (Elliot et al 1997). The amputation was oblique with extra skin on the ulnar side of the stump; the stump was closed with a skin graft. This left him with absence of his left, non-dominant

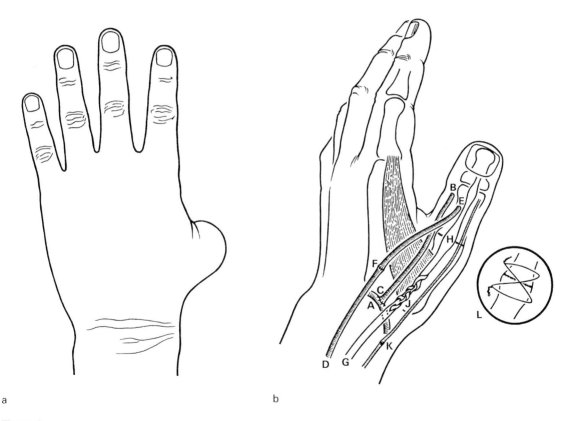

a   b

Figure 9

(a) Preoperative thumb stump. (b) The surgical 'hook-up' (by courtesy of K Harrison). A, radial a.; B, dorsalis pedis a.; C, radial a. – dorsalis pedis a. anastomosed; D, cephalic v.; E, dorsal v.; F, cephalic v, – dorsal v. anastomosed; G, extensor pollicis longus t.; H, extensor hallucis longus t.; J, extensor pollicis longus t. – extensor hallucis longus t. woven; K, dorsal n. anastomosed; L, osteosynthesis.

thumb, which meant he could not play the chanter pipe of his bagpipes. He was offered a reconstruction with a hallux transfer (Buncke et al 1973, O'Brien et al 1975). He was shown patients who had had such a transfer and was able to make his own decision about whether this was a reconstruction that would allow him to get back to being a professional musician.

A left hallux transfer for left thumb reconstruction was performed. At surgery the left hallux was taken through the metatarsal phalangeal joint. The dorsalis pedis artery and its metatarsal continuation was taken for the arterial input and the dorsal venous system for the venous drainage. Both the volar digital nerves and a dorsal sensory nerve were taken. The flexor hallucis longus and extensor hallucis longus were taken for later repair. The foot was closed primarily with preservation of the head of the first metatarsal ray.

The toe was attached with a metacarpophalangeal joint arthrodesis. Flexor and extensor tendon repairs to power the interphalangeal joint were performed and three nerves were repaired. The arthrodesis was performed with two parallel k-wires and a figure of eight compression wire. The dorsalis pedis artery was anastomosed end to side to the radial artery in the anatomical snuffbox and the venous drainage to the cephalic vein (see Fig. 9b). The transfer went without complications and the osteosynthesis site healed primarily. Much care was taken to ensure the osteosynthesis was correctly placed to give optimal positioning of the thumb pulp. The reconstructed thumb had a basal joint and an interphalangeal joint and the arthrodesis was performed with the right amount of flexion and a little rotation so it could be optimally placed on the A-hole of the chanter pipe.

He began playing his pipes at 3 months postoperatively. The thumb has retained full carpometacarpal joint movement and has 30° of interphalangeal joint range of movement. Sensory return is such that he can feel the opening of the A-hole with his reconstructed thumb pulp. The measured static 2-point discrimination on the reconstructed thumb is 14 mm and on the opposite toe, which has not been moved, 11 mm.

The only problem he had in his rehabilitation is that he developed ingrowing of the thumb nail and had to undergo a resection 3 mm on both

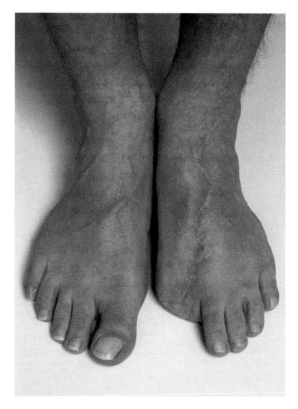

Figure 10

Donor toe defect.

sides of the germinal matrix of the new thumb nail to prevent this ingrowing.

Surgical result

See Figs 10–14.

Discussion

The deficit in the musician's function must be assessed carefully. He or she must then be given all the reconstructive options. In a complex reconstruction like a toe transfer the musician should be shown patients who have had such a transfer to provide the information necessary to

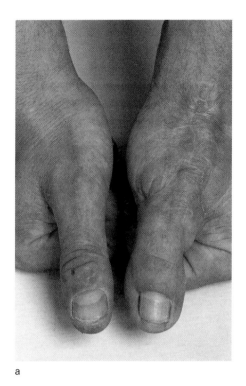

a

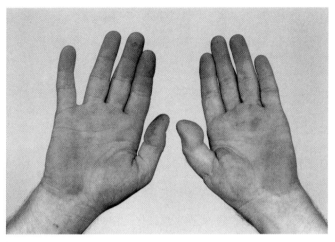

b

Figure 11

Healed toe-to-thumb transfer. (a) Dorsal view: note the scar over the anatomical snuffbox at the site of the microvascular anastomoses. (b) Palmar view: note the slightly increased bulk of toe pulp.

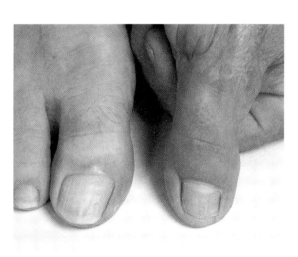

Figure 12

'Thumb' nail narrowed surgically to prevent ingrowing and improve cosmesis. The reconstruction is shown in comparison to the intact right hallux.

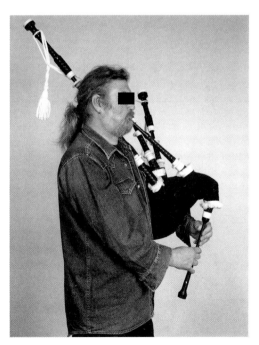

Figure 13

The patient playing.

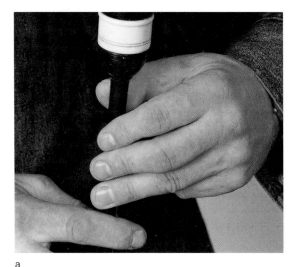

a

Figure 14

(a, b) Detail of the left thumb on the chanter. Note the thumb is active in fingering the A-hole.

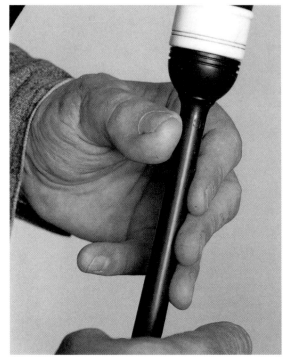

b

make a personal decision about which of the complex reconstructions is the best.

Such a complex reconstruction needs to be performed by a surgical team who are well practised in the management of it. In such a specialized area, where the reconstruction is so valuable and unique, it must be done by a surgical team with a great deal of expertise. This will involve sending patients to different units and this should be actively encouraged.

Case report 2

Scapholunate dissociation in association with a severe wrist fracture in a professional pianist

John Stanley

Although musicians suffer from specific problems engendered by the demands made of them by their particular talent and instrument, they are not immune from injuries that occur in ordinary life. However, the high level of manual dexterity required by musicians places additional responsibilities on surgeons or physicians when dealing with what might be regarded as 'ordinary' trauma.

In particular those injuries which occur in and around the hand and wrist, on either the dominant or non-dominant side, often have a profound effect upon the capacity of the musician to play at the previously attained high standard. Therefore, it is extremely important fully to evaluate the injuries and perhaps more importantly specifically to determine the prognosis.

The prognosis does not include only what the wrist or hand will be like in 1, 2, 5 or 10 years but how long it is going to take to recover from the injury and what specific impairment or disability is likely to accrue. Therefore, a realistic appraisal of the treatment options, the rehabilitation and retraining requirements and the time taken to recover from the injury is an essential part of the discussion with the individual.

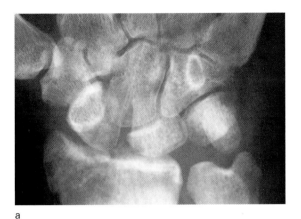

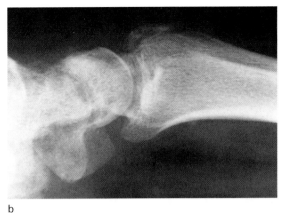

a   b

Figure 15

X-rays, (a) anteroposterior and (b) lateral magnified, of the injured wrist showing the die punch fracture and scapholunate dissociation and collapse of the scaphoid (the ring sign).

Patient

A 26-year-old pianist of concert standard, sustained a complex injury to his carpus with an associated intra-articular fracture of his distal radius as a result of a fall. This trans-styloid lesser arc injury to the right dominant wrist was treated primarily with percutaneous pinning of the Chauffeur fracture, but the intercarpal ligament injury between the scaphoid and the lunate and between the triquetrum and the lunate was not recognized and treated at the initial surgical procedure. This resulted in a rotary instability of the scaphoid and the classic collapse deformity seen in these cases (Linscheid et al 1972, Mayfield 1984) (Fig. 15). Other instability patterns may present, such as ulnar mid-carpal instability (Lichtman et al 1981), and require specific investigation and evaluation (usually arthroscopic examination) (Kelly and Stanley 1990) and if appropriate arthroscopic surgery (Stanley and Saffar 1994). As a result of the ensuing severe restriction of motion he was referred 5 months from the original injury for further treatment in the form of a ligament reconstruction to the right scapholunate interosseous ligament.

The treatment options for this young man were dictated by his need to be able to play a keyboard or piano at a very high level. This requires 30° of flexion and 30° of extension, 15° of ulnar deviation and 5° of radial deviation of the wrist. Rotary instability of the scaphoid indicates that the lateral column of the wrist has collapsed into its default position; that is to say, it flexes until it can flex no more. This has the net effect of restricting any further flexion of the wrist at the radiocarpal joint, and therefore the only flexion that is available is via the mid-carpal joint. However, the lunate in its collapsed (extended) position falls into full extension so that it cannot extend any more; thus any extension that occurs at the wrist level can only occur at the mid-carpal joint level, but this is already restricted by excess scaphoid flexion and so a considerable loss of range of motion in flexion and extension is inevitable and did occur in this case. (His active and passive range of wrist motion in all planes prior to reconstruction was zero.)

Perhaps more importantly, in patients with very mobile scaphoid bones, radial deviation and ulnar deviation is normally accompanied by significant flexion and extension (Craigen and Stanley 1995) and translation of the scaphoid (Fig. 16), and, of course, the triquetrum translates and rotates. In the collapse deformity (dorsal intercalated segmental instability, DISI) occasioned by scapholunate interosseous ligament rupture and

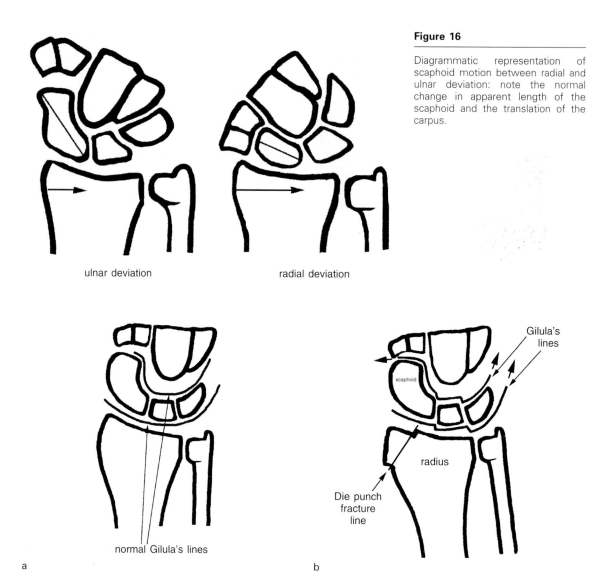

ulnar deviation   radial deviation

Figure 16

Diagrammatic representation of scaphoid motion between radial and ulnar deviation: note the normal change in apparent length of the scaphoid and the translation of the carpus.

normal Gilula's lines

Gilula's lines

scaphoid

Die punch fracture line

radius

a   b

Figure 17

(a, b) Diagrammatic representation of Gilula's lines.

perilunate ligament injuries, the capacity for radial and ulnar deviation is also severely restricted, clearly a point of crucial importance to musicians and in particular to concert standard pianists.

The X-rays in Fig. 15 show the characteristic signet ring sign of the scaphoid, the previous die punch fracture of the radial styloid and the Terry Thomas sign, that is, the gap between the scaphoid and the lunate. Perhaps more importantly from a diagnostic point of view is the apparent break in Gilula's lines; these lines are drawn along the mid-carpal joint and form a continuous unbroken line on the capitate surface of the scaphoid and the lunate and the hamate surface of the triquetrum (Fig. 17). Like Shenton's line of the hip, this line is meant to be unbroken.

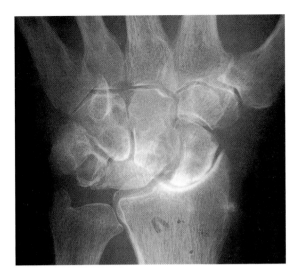

Figure 18

An X-ray of a wrist with the SLAC (scapholunate advanced collapse) pattern degeneration.

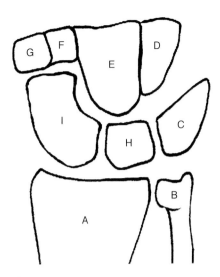

Figure 19

Diagrammatic representation of the columns of the wrist. A, radius; B, ulna; C, triquetrum; D, hamate; E, capitate; F, trapezoid; G, trapezium; H, lunate; I, scaphoid. C = medial column of wrist; DEFGH = central column of wrist, I = lateral column of wrist.

It can be seen from Fig. 15 that they are indeed broken, indicating both scapholunate and triquetrolunate ligament injury: in fact, this the classic lesser arc injury described by Mayfield (Mayfield 1984).

The treatment protocol for these patients is determined by the available surgical options and by the symptom level of the patient, but it is widely accepted that if completely untreated this degree of injury will almost certainly result in eventual degenerative arthrosis of the scapholunate advanced collapse pattern (SLAC) described by Kirk Watson and his group. (Fig. 18) (Watson et al 1986).

Surgical options

The surgical options are in reality quite stark when one is faced with a chronic collapse situation. Either some form of soft tissue reconstruction is performed or an intercarpal arthrodesis is chosen. The term 'chronic' indicates that one would determine that injuries over 12 months would have significant secondary changes to make the likelihood of a primary repair of the

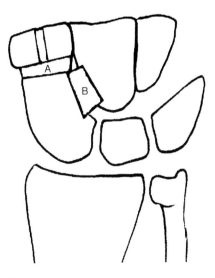

Figure 20

Diagrammatic representation of scaphotrapezioltrapezoidal arthrodesis (A) and scaphocapitate arthrodesis (B).

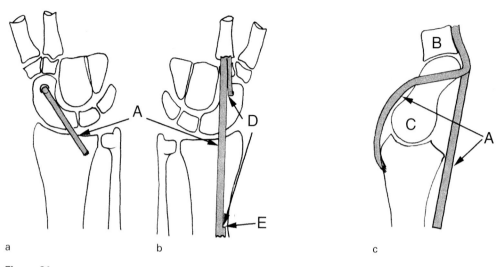

a   b   c

Figure 21

Diagrammatic representation of the Brunelli procedure: (a) dosal, (b) volar and (c) lateral aspects. A, flexor carpi radialis; B, trapezium; C, scaphoid; D, tendon stripped to here from here; E, tendon harvested from here.

damaged ligament extremely difficult or in the majority of cases impossible.

The intercarpal fusions described for this condition are either stabilization of the lateral (scaphoid) column or stabilization of the central (lunate) column of the wrist (Fig. 19).

Stabilization of the lateral column involves either a scapho-trapezio-trapezoidal (STT) arthrodesis, as described by Kirk Watson (Watson et al 1986), or a scaphocapitate arthrodesis (Fig. 20). The former has been shown by Kleinman (Kleinman and Carroll 1990) and others to have good medium to long-term results but modest or poor results at 5 years (Rogers and Watson 1989) with the development of posterior rim arthrosis (Vender et al 1987). Scaphocapitate fusion appears to reduce the risk but as the mechanics of this arthrodesis are only slightly different from those of STT arthrodesis, it is likely that a group of patients will develop secondary arthrosis from this procedure also in the fullness of time.

If, as is described above, it is inappropriate to perform a primary repair of the scapholunate interosseous ligament because of the time interval since injury (Stanley and Trail 1994), then two procedures are currently available. The first, described by Blatt (Blatt 1987), is the dorsal capsulodesis which involves providing a dorsal tether to the scaphoid preventing its collapse. The second is the Brunelli (Brunelli and Brunelli 1995) procedure, which involves using flexor carpi radialis tendon in part to reinforce the scapho-trapezial ligament (the ligament of Kuhlmann) (Boabighi et al 1993) and passing through the drill hole in the scaphoid to the dorsal aspect of the wrist, crossing the scapholunate interval, thus reinforcing this area (Fig. 21).

Our own figures for both these procedures show that with procedures performed in the period from 6 months to 18 months following injury the results of surgery are good in the medium and long term. However, for the Blatt procedure we have found that a delay of 3 years or more before the institution of appropriate treatment results in a high dissatisfaction rate, almost certainly due to chronic capsular contracture preventing adequate correction.

The ideal (Stanley and Trail 1994) is to recognize at the outset that ligament injuries can and do occur in isolation but inevitably arise as a result of die punch (axial depression) fractures of the scaphoid or lunate fossa. These injuries require serious consideration for accurate fracture reduction (arthroscopically assisted), including possible direct repair of the interosseous ligament posteriorly. The results of early treatment of ligament injuries by direct repair are extremely encouraging and give rise to a minimal loss of long-term function. In the case of the subacute injury, that is, up to and including 4 months, primary repair remains the procedure of choice. Primary repair must always be accompanied by temporary fixation of the scaphoid to the capitate and to the lunate with Kirschner wires for a period of a minimum of 6 weeks and preferably 8 weeks. Delayed primary repair and secondary reconstructions also require this period of immobilization.

Surgical results

This patient gained significant wrist motion in association with loss of wrist pain and synovitis following the Brunelli reconstruction. He was able to resume limited playing 4 months following repair (9 months from initial injury) and achieved full playing potential 4 months later. His wrist motion (after extensive hand therapy) at that time was recorded as flexion 60°, extension 55°, ulnar deviation 30°, radial deviation 10°. He was about to resume a music scholarship he had won before his accident.

The results of surgery for significant intercarpal injury of the type described above recover well within 4–5 months but cannot be adequately assessed in less than 12 months; the rehabilitation of these patients can take up to 18 months, and improvement in functional capacity can be seen up to 2 years. An apparent improvement in function is often obtained by adaptation of playing technique, which may involve some technical deterioration, but it is clear that if this is occurring, careful monitoring of the technique by a teacher is essential and almost mandatory in order to ensure that poor technique does not become 'the norm', with all the attendant problems of the 'knock on' effect so often seen in musicians who have had to adapt their previously good technique to accommodate for injury and loss of facility.

Case report 3

Secondary flexor tendon grafting in a 70-year-old violinist

Ian Winspur

Secondary reconstruction

Even under ideal circumstances, injury or damage to important structures may only present after the 'golden period' for primary repair has passed. This is unfortunate, for secondary reconstruction is usually less predictable than primary repair and indeed may carry additional risks to non-damaged structures. However, when dealing with a musician in whom even a 1% fall-off in performance may not be compatible with professional playing, efforts put into secondary reconstruction will generally be well rewarded.

Secondary reconstruction usually requires very precise and specific postoperative hand therapy and the musician is usually well motivated and sufficiently well co-ordinated to be able to co-operate and comply completely. Therefore, as a general rule, it is worth embarking upon secondary reconstruction in the musician even when relative contraindications exist. This of course is contrary to current wisdom, which perceives musicians in general as poor candidates for surgery. The following case illustrates the complexity but the value of secondary reconstruction in the musician.

Patient

A 70-year-old active amateur violinist sustained a small but deep laceration with a kitchen knife over the flexor aspect of his left (fingering) index finger immediately proximal to the PIP joint crease. He was seen in the local casualty department where he was examined and the wound sutured. It was felt at the time that active flexion of the finger was present and that therefore the flexor tendons were intact. However, over the next 2 weeks finger flexion became increasingly more difficult and suddenly 2 weeks after injury the patient found himself completely unable to flex either the DIP or PIP joints and only with very limited flexion at the metaphalangeal (MP) joints. He sought help from his GP and was referred to the specialist 6 weeks after the original injury with clear evidence of complete division of both flexor tendons to his left index finger. The digital nerves were intact. The patient was devastated as his playing career seemed at an end.

Surgical options

1. No treatment and acceptance of the functional loss
2. Attempted reconstruction of the flexor mechanism of the index finger by free-tendon grafting either in one or two stages.

Option 1 was not acceptable to the patient. Therefore, option 2 was the only alternative.

Contraindications

This elderly patient had huge puffy hands and early osteoarthritis in the distal joints. There was therefore a significant chance of his developing gross stiffness in the rest of his undamaged hand and indeed also of being left with a stiff flexed index finger. With osteoarthritis already present in the distal joint of the index finger, the chances of obtaining the active 50° of DIP flexion required to finger the E-string on his violin were slim. Tender scarring to the pulp and the tip of the finger either due to the basic surgical incision or from punctate scar from through-and-through suturing of the distal tendon graft stump would also preclude playing.

Surgical reconstruction (measurement and fine tuning)

On careful analysis preoperatively it was found that the index finger in this man's case required 90° of flexion at the MP joint, 90° of flexion at the PIP joint and 50° of flexion at the DIP joint to be able to touch the E-string on the violin. Surgery was performed under local anaesthesia and at exploration it was found that the profundus and sublimis had been completely divided at the level of the A3 pulley in no man's land

and the proximal stumps had retracted into the palm. The A3 pulley was destroyed, but the rest of the flexor sheath was pristine. Therefore, a palmaris longus graft was harvested and inserted from the proximal profundus stump at the level of the lumbrical origin to the distal profundus stump without using through-and-through pulp tip sutures. The sublimis tendon was resected at the level of the carpal tunnel. Protected active motion was started on the fourth postoperative day. Recovery of motion was slow, but 16 weeks following surgery 90° of active MP and 90° of active PIP flexion had been obtained with near full extension of the digit. However, only 10° of active DIP flexion could be obtained to provide a total DIP flexion of 20°, 30° short of that required to finger the E-string. In view of the excellent active motion already obtained at the proximal joints, a decision was taken to fuse the distal joint in the required playing position, which was again accurately measured at 50° of flexion. Compression arthrodesis (Allende and Engleman 1980) was performed 20 weeks following grafting, measuring the position of the arthrodesis carefully at surgery and using a single k-wire and dorsal compression band technique (see Chapter 7). Because of skin tension due to the extremely flexed position of the distal phalanx and the need to preserve bone length, dorsal advancement skin flaps had to be utilized during closure. Primary healing ensued, however, and the patient was allowed to start limited practice on the violin 6 weeks from arthrodesis. The axial pin was removed 6 weeks later. The patient began practice playing 7 months from injury and at 12 months from injury was starting to play again publicly. His only difficulty, at that point, he stated, was with the technically demanding occasional need for 'double stopping'; he was able to 'double stop' after the tertiary procedure.

Surgical result

(See Figs 22–27).

Discussion

One would not normally commit a 70-year-old man with division of both flexor tendons in his

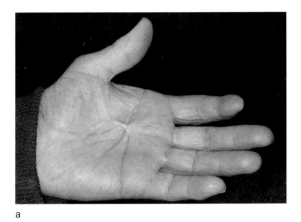

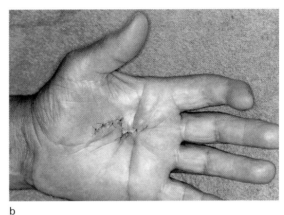

a

b

Figure 22

(a) A 70-year-old violinist 8 months after secondary flexor tendon reconstruction of his left index finger by free tendon grafting and dorsal interphalangeal arthrodesis; the hand in extension; (b) the contracted scar was released as a tertiary procedure.

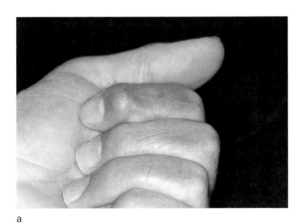

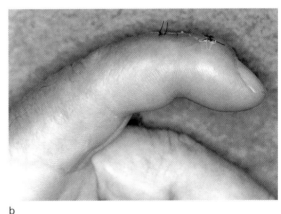

a

b

Figure 23

(a) The hand in flexion; the dorsal skin is still inflamed due to the presence of tension wire. (b) The tension wire was then removed as a tertiary procedure.

non-dominant index finger to a 7-month secondary flexor tendon reconstruction. Indeed, the reconstruction would be contraindicated in normal circumstances. However, in this man's case with the determination fostered by complete despair at loss of his playing ability, the long road proved to be worthwhile. As it transpired, the distal joint did not flex actively to the required degree and required arthrodesis in the playing position. However, this in itself was a minor technical piece of fine tuning and worked extremely satisfactorily.

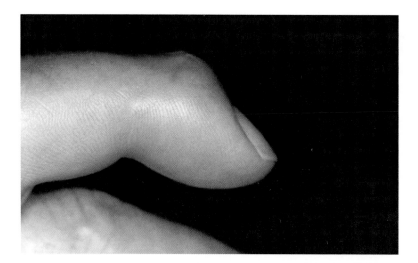

Figure 24

The position of dorsal interphalangeal arthrodesis calculated to allow fingering of the E-string on the violin.

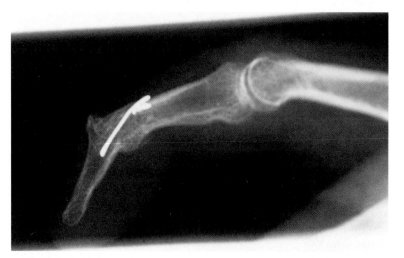

Figure 25

Healed arthrodesis with tension band wire still in place (later removed).

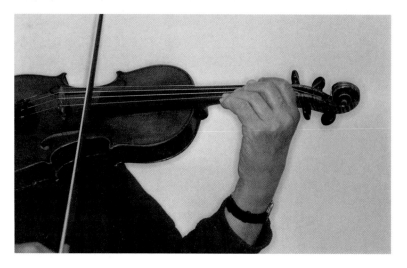

Figure 26

Patient playing 8 months after start of reconstruction.

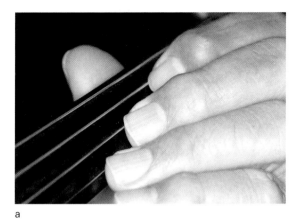 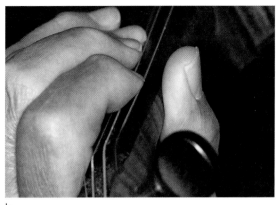

a   b

Figure 27

(a, b) The position of the index fingertip on the violin.

Case report 4

Secondary reconstruction by surgical releases and skin grafting

Stewart Watson

Patient

The patient was a 40-year-old right-handed professional Country and Western guitarist, who while staying in a London hotel several years ago after a concert woke up with what he thought was an insect bite. Within an hour the dorsum of his left hand was swelling and red; within 3 hours he was in a hyperbaric oxygen chamber; and within another few hours the skin was sloughing off the back of his hand (Snyder and Leonard 1990).

On investigation it was found that the hotel was frequented by Australian students, many in transit. Venomous spiders and these types of injury are seen in Australia, but are unusual in Britain where poisonous spiders currently do not naturally exist.

The patient underwent several skin grafting operations; a surgical attempt was also made to provide coverage by a distant skin flap from the outer aspect of his arm, but this also failed. Eight weeks after the initial bite, the hand was still unhealed and, despite continuous hand therapy, very stiff, contracted and deformed. The original wounds were still open (Fig. 28). Mycobacterium (not uncommon in spider venom) (Oppenheimer and Taggart 1990) was cultured in the wound, so further delaying healing and surgical reconstruction.

Surgical options

Two options existed: to achieve coverage and accept stiffness or to embark on surgical complete release and coverage by high-quality skin grafts, with a massive postoperative hand therapy regime. The first option was not acceptable to the patient.

Surgical result

Formal surgical excision and releases were therefore performed 4 months from the original injury (Fig. 29). Complete coverage was obtained by thick partial-thickness skin grafts. Hand therapy was restarted immediately. At this stage, the wounds were unhealed and required frequent dressings; movement in the hand was very limited and as healing progressed slowly, the resultant scarring

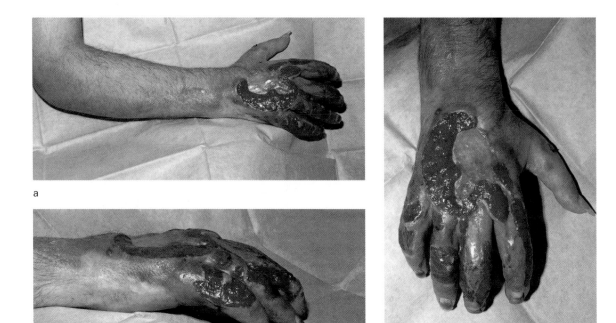

a

b

c

Figure 28

(a, b, c) Patient's hand, 4 months after a bite by a venomous spider, with persisting open wounds, swelling and gross deformity. Remnants of healed skin graft and failed flap are visible.

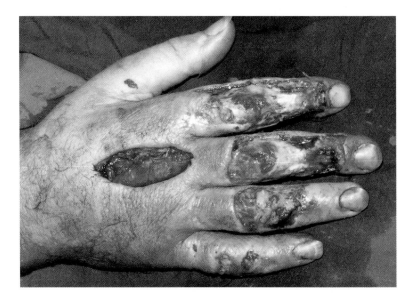

Figure 29

Intra-operative photograph after surgical release and excision of unhealthy wound and scar. Note complete release has been achieved.

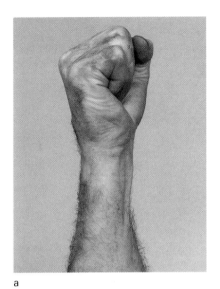

a

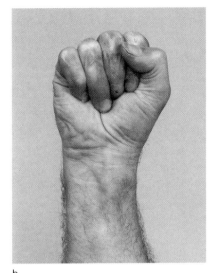

b

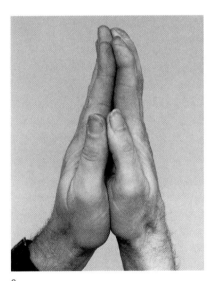

c

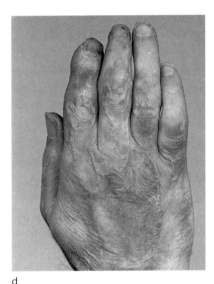

d

Figure 30

(a,b,c,d) Final result: excellent mobility, sufficient to play Country and Western guitar professionally.

was hypertrophic and contracted. Hand therapy was administered three times each week for the first 6 months, taking the form of dorsal serial splintage to increase the metacarpophalangeal joint flexion, the application of flexion devices, prolonged passive stretching and activities against resistance (including guitar playing!).

Pressure garments were applied early, before wound healing, with the aid of hydrocolloid dressings, to assist oedema reduction and for scar management. As movement returned, so frequency of treatment reduced and the hand achieved a full active range of motion 18 months from the time of injury (Fig. 30).

The patient was under hand therapy care for 18 months, with two sessions daily as an inpatient for 2 weeks, three sessions weekly for 6 months, and one session weekly for 12 months. His complete recovery took 2 years, but he has resumed playing and a full professional career.

Discussion

The surgical techniques used to salvage this patient's hand are basic. Compression garments and gloves are essential in controlling scar hypertrophy and swelling. However, only a highly motivated patient can sustain a long course of therapy, and this patient's excellent final result was largely attributable to his high level of determination to return to his profession. The fact that his surgeons were prepared to go the extra mile only laid the foundation for his final recovery.

The spider, incidentally, was believed to have been of the Australian White Tip variety.

References

Allende B, Engleman J (1980) Tension band arthrodesis in finger joints. *J Hand Surg Am* **5**:269–71.

Amadio PC (1995) Open reduction of intra-articular fractures of the distal radius. In: Saffar P, Cooney WP, eds. *Fractures of the Distal Radius*. Martin Dunitz: London: 193–202.

Blatt G (1987) Capsulodesis in reconstructive hand surgery: dorsal capsulodesis for the unstable scaphoid and volar capsulodesis following excision of the distal ulna. *Hand Clin* **3**:81–102.

Boabighi A, Kuhlmann JN, Kenesi C (1993) The distal ligamentous complex of the scaphoid and the scapholunate ligament. An anatomical, histological and biomechanical study. *J Hand Surg Br* **18**:65–9.

Brunelli Georgio A, Brunelli Giovanni R (1995) A new technique to correct carpal instability with scaphoid rotary subluxation: preliminary report. *J Hand Surg Am* **20A**(3, Part 2):S82–5.

Buncke HJ, McLean DH, George PT (1973) Thumb replacement: great toe transplantation by microvascular anastomosis. *Br J Plast Surg* **26**:194.

Craigen MA, Stanley JK (1995) Wrist kinematics. Row, column or both? *J Hand Surg Br* **20**:165–70.

Crawford GP (1976) Screw fixation for certain fractures of the phalanges and metacarpals. *J Bone Joint Surg Am* **58**:487–92.

Crawford GP (1984) Polythene splints for mallet finger deformities. *J Hand Surg Am* **9**:231–7.

Elliot D Sood MK, Fleming AFS, Swain B (1997) A comparison of replantation and terminalisation after distal finger amputation. *J Hand Surg Br* **22**:523–9.

Kelly EP, Stanley JK (1990) Arthroscopy of the wrist. *J Hand Surg Br* **15**:236–42.

Kleinman WB, Carroll C 4th (1990) Scapho-trapezio-trapezoid arthrodesis for treatment of chronic static and dynamic scapho-lunate instability: a 10 year perspective on pitfalls and complications. *J Hand Surg Am* **15**(3):408–14.

Leddy J (1993) Flexor tendons – acute injury. In: Green D, ed. *Operative Hand Surgery*, vol. 2. (3rd edn). Churchill Livingstone: New York: 1823–45.

Lichtman DM, Schneider JR, Swafford AR, Mack GR (1981) Ulnar midcarpal instability – clinical and laboratory analysis. *J Hand Surg Am* **6**:515–23.

Linscheid RL, Dobyns JH, Beabout JW, Bryan RS (1972) Traumatic instability of the wrist. Diagnosis, classification and pathomechanics. *J Bone Joint Surg Am* **54**:1612–32.

Mayfield JK (1984) Patterns of injury to carpal ligaments. A spectrum. *Clin Orthop* **187**:36–42.

O'Brien GM, MacLeod AM, Sykes PJ et al (1975) Hallux-to-hand transfer. *Hand* **7**:128.

Oppenheimer B, Taggart I (1990) More in spider venom than venom? *The Lancet* **335**:228.

Rogers WD, Watson HK (1989) Radial styloid impingement after triscaphe arthrodesis. *J Hand Surg Am* **14**(2, Part 1):297–301.

Snyder C, Leonard L (1990) Bites and stings of the hands. In: Tubiana R, ed. *The Hand*, vol. 3. WB Saunders: Philadelphia: 873–902.

Stanley JK, Saffar P (1994) *Wrist Arthroscopy*. Martin Dunitz: London.

Stanley JK, Trail IA (1994) Carpal instability. *J Bone Joint Surg Br* **76**:691–700.

Vender MI, Watson HK, Wiener BD, Black DM (1987) Degenerative change in symptomatic scaphoid nonunion. *J Hand Surg Am* **12**:514–19.

Watson HK, Ryu J, Akelman E (1986) Limited triscaphoid intercarpal arthrodesis for rotatory subluxation of the scaphoid. *J Bone Joint Surg Am* **68**:345–9.

Wilgis EFS, Brushart TM (1993) Nerve repair and grafting. In: Green DP, ed. *Operative Hand Surgery*, vol. 2. (3rd edn). Churchill Livingstone: New York: 1315–40.

Wilson AJ, Mann FA, Gilula LA (1990) Imaging the hand and wrist. *J Hand Surg Br* **15**(2):153–67.

Winspur I (1983) Fingertip injuries. In: Boswick JA, ed. *Current Concepts in Hand Surgery*. Lea and Febiger: Philadelphia: 19–23.

Zancolli EA (1979) Pathology of the extensor apparatus of the finger. In: Zancolli EA, *The Structural and Dynamic Basis of Hand Surgery*. JB Lippincott: Philadelphia: 79–902.

11

The physical therapist's contribution

Hand

Alison T Davis and Gabriele Rogers

Musicians are a unique group of people with very specific requirements from their hands. Years of practice will have given them very precise control and co-ordination to achieve mastery at their chosen instrument. Any damage to the musculoskeletal system, whether by injury or necessary surgery, will affect this special mobility. This mobility needs to be regained to an exact requirement by the musician working with the hand therapist during the rehabilitation phase following injury or surgery (Fig. 1).

Assessment

Prior to embarking upon any treatment regime, a thorough and careful examination by the hand therapist is essential. Problems can be identified and discussed and measurements can be taken and recorded. The musician's comments about the musical instrument concerned can be of particular value, especially if the therapist is unfamiliar with that particular instrument. The therapist should also be aware of any relevant past history and have details of any treatment so far provided. The therapist should also be aware of any medication the musician is taking, particularly steroids and beta blockers (see Chapter 17).

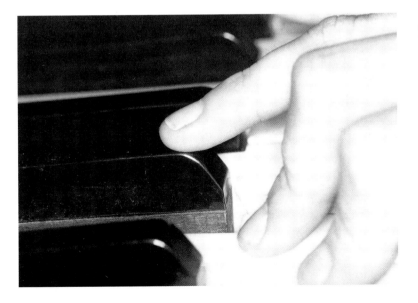

Figure 1

The excursion of the fingertip required to move from white to black keys on the piano = 16–17 mm.

A detailed musical history is also important and the following questions should be considered.

- Is the musician still able to play his instrument correctly or is he being forced into compromised posture and technique to maintain performance?
- Is the musician able to play at all, and if so, for how long?
- Has there been any change or alteration in daily practice patterns or in the demands of the actual musical repertoire?
- Has the musician's playing environment changed?
- Has the conductor changed, the playing partner or the seating position been altered?

It is also essential that the therapist be aware of the risk factors imposed by that musician's particular instrument, either through the necessary playing posture, the speed and nature of the movements required to play the instrument or the strength of muscles required to support the instrument while playing. Additionally, the therapist should be aware of the stresses and strains placed on the musician's physique when transporting large, cumbersome instruments, such as the double bass, from place to place.

When examining the musician, particular note should be taken of the overall body posture and playing posture with the patient undressed. To achieve this the musician must always be observed in his playing posture, both in a static position and in his active playing position. It is also important to note the relative importance of each joint necessary for musical performance in each patient since, for example, a stiff shoulder or painful neck can severely affect a violinist, but have much less effect on a pianist, whereas a diminished span, secondary to hand or joint contracture, can significantly affect a pianist, while having little effect on a violinist. Routine palpation, assessment and recording of the range of movement of joints and recording of muscle strength is standard. Proximal joints must also be included and sensory changes are also noted and recorded. Postural problems and decreased range of motion can be addressed and corrected by skilled therapists, but identification and correction of poor technique can usually only be achieved by a skilled music teacher and often a multidisciplinary assessment, taking more than one session, is required.

Practical methods of measurement

Standard, easily reproducible methods of measurement are essential for the results to be meaningful and valuable. From the patient's point of view there is a great psychological boost on seeing measurable improvement. For the therapist, accurate measurements are required at all stages in treatment to evaluate the effectiveness of treatment.

A small goniometer is used to measure joint range in the fingers. The goniometer is used over the dorsum of the fingers and using a scale of 0° for full extension and 90°+ for full flexion. All joints in the area of injury are routinely measured. However, total excursion of a digit is also important and this is more easily measured as distance from a fixed point. The commonest and most useful measurements are:

- Tip of finger to distal palmar crease
- Elevation of fingertip from a flat surface (Fig. 2)
- Direct measure of thumb/index web span, or any interdigital web span
- Thumb rotation to adjacent identified digit metaphalangeal (MP) crease.

Grip strength and pinch are measured on the standard commercially available dynamometers. The musician is also taught simple practical measurement with a ruler so he can monitor his own progress and set limited goals during unsupervised home therapy.

Modalities of treatment

Standard modalities of treatment are utilized. They are:

- Ice and elevation
- Compression
- Electrotherapy
- Massage
- Splinting
- Exercise.

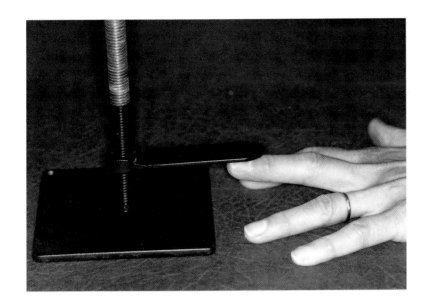

Figure 2

Threaded device to monitor, strengthen and increase critical finger extension in a pianist.

In treating injury, early treatment is aimed at reducing oedema, inflammation and pain and preventing further injury. Ice, elevation and rest are encouraged, together with non-steroidal anti-inflammatory medication. As soon as the acute phase has passed the emphasis changes, particularly with musicians, with gentle graded exercises often consisting only of gentle shadow playing or light playing on the instrument for 4- to 5-minute sessions twice or thrice a day to encourage early mobility. Protective, supportive splinting or taping may be required, but practising on the instrument is encouraged. As the patient's discomfort diminishes and motion and strength develop, the patient is then placed on a graded work (music) hardening programme, increasing the 4- to 5-minute playing sessions twice or thrice a day to four to six times a day and increasing the duration in a stepwise fashion every 3–4 days. Chronic problems can be similarly treated and part of the treatment programme must include conditioning and preventive measures to reduce the risk of reinjury.

Ice and elevation are an effective method of reducing oedema following injury or surgery. It is of paramount importance to reduce oedema quickly and effectively, for it in itself can lead to increasing pain and movement restrictions and persisting oedema can cause the development of tissue fibrosis. Ice baths for a few minutes or ice compresses locally cause vasoconstriction, so reducing oedema. Contrast baths improve circulation generally, so aiding oedema dispersal. The hand is alternately immersed in bowls of hot and cold water for 1–3 minutes at a time for up to 15 or 20 minutes, starting and ending in hot water. Elevation is critical to oedema dispersal, and in the early postoperative period high elevation with the hand held on the top of the head, unless when resting, when it is propped on pillows, greatly reduces oedema and pain and facilitates early mobilization. Compression will also aid oedema dispersal. Tubigrip, Lycra finger stalls, Coban wrap and rubber bandage wrapping are all effective means of applying pressure. Intermittent pressure can also be applied with a pneumatic cuff (pneumotherapy). Massage, especially effleurage and gentle kneading will also decrease oedema, but it is time-consuming. Controlled active movement, if permissible, will also squeeze oedema fluid from the tissues if combined with high elevation.

The various heat modalities all aid in mobilization by improving circulation, reducing inflammation, softening tissues and easing pain. The heat can be applied by moist heat packs and warm hand soaks. All have to be supervised carefully as inflamed and injured tissues are more susceptible to burn injury than normal tissues.

It is also important to note that ultrasound may not be used if the patient is taking steroids or if a steroid injection has been administered within 7 days. Ultrasound is a very effective modality for decreasing inflammation but care must be taken in its application.

Following healing, early gentle scar massage with soft cream is very beneficial in helping to reduce and align collagen formation and reduce rigid scar formation. The patient is taught self-massage. It is also important that the musician, normally so impatient, fully understands the nature of scar maturing and softening and understands the biological timeframes involved in this process. Otherwise despondency will develop when slight restriction is still present due to scar immaturity, as long as 4–6 months after the injury.

Splinting for the musician's hand

External splintage can be utilized to provide protection and support for injured or healing structures, but it can also be utilized as a tool to help regain mobility in joints or gliding structures with reduced range of motion. The subject of splinting is vast. The fundamental concepts and principles are meticulously covered by Fess and Phillips (1987). Splinting has developed considerably over the last 20 years with the development of new low-temperature thermoplastic materials. The basic choice of materials initially was between perforated or unperforated plastic (Fig. 3). Now the hand therapist can choose between drape and rigidity, between thick or thin, between plastics with or without memory, between self-bonding or non, and has a choice of colours (see Appendix II for a list of thermoplastics and their individual properties). The advantages of low-temperature thermoplastics over plaster of Paris and even fibreglass are the increased precision allowed from their malleability and readjustability. Splints, so constructed, can also be designed to be strong yet removable, so allowing the patient to bathe or allowing limited unsupported exercise to the part, if appropriate, thereby enabling earlier

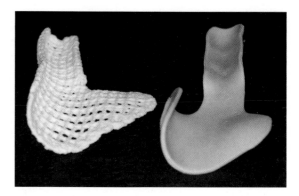

Figure 3

Perforated and unperforated thermoplastic splints.

mobilization to take place. The thermoplastics themselves can be cleaned, thus aiding hygiene, which is important with early postoperative wounds. They are also aesthetically pleasing and fixation, generally with Velcro straps, makes application simple. Their precisely mouldable properties make it much easier to provide precision support to areas which need it, but to leave unaffected joints unrestricted.

Patients can return to some physical activities earlier by wearing thermoplastic splints to provide some protection. This is important for musicians as early return to their musical instrument is often possible with the protection of a custom-moulded splint (Figs 4 and 5).

The musician's afflictions often relate to coincidental injury or accidents frequently associated with sport or DIY (home improvements). But in certain circumstances their symptoms relate entirely to their musical activity and the instrument they play. Specific playing-related problems are:

- Synovitis of overstressed joints
- Synovitis of the carpometacarpal (CMC) joint of the thumb, due to excessive power pinch or loading
- Chronic painful synovitis of the interphalangeal (IP) joint of the thumb in woodwind players due to taking the weight of the instrument
- Aggravation of a painful pre-existing arthritis in a joint while playing.

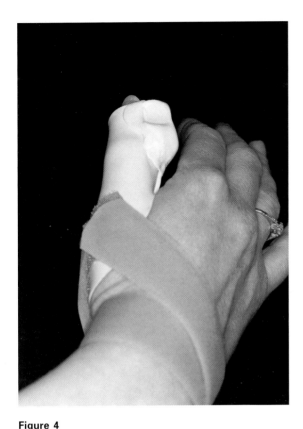

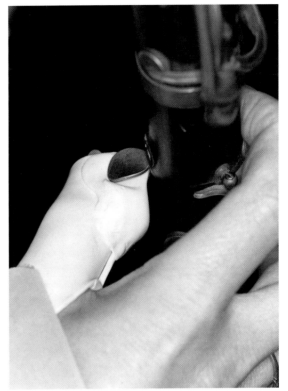

Figure 4

Temporary supportive splint.

Figure 5

The splint enables early return to playing following thumb IP joint injury.

The principal non-playing related conditions seen are:

- Proximal interphalangeal (PIP) injuries and sprains
- Finger fractures
- Extensor and flexor tendon injuries
- Wrist and scaphoid fractures and intercarpal ligament injuries
- Postoperative cases.

Although some of the instrument-related problems can be alleviated through changes in technique or to the instrument itself, the affected joints may require temporary rest and protective splinting whilst playing. This is where joint splintage, which can easily be performed with thermoplastic splinting, can be of great benefit. In the management of post-traumatic rehabilitation the strength and removability of external supportive thermoplastic splints can be utilized to great advantage to allow unresisted active motion intermittently at a very early stage and even to allow 'shadow playing' or very light finger exercises on the instrument at an early point with the splint removed.

In a chronic painful synovitis of the IP joint of the thumb in woodwind players when the weight of the instrument is being taken on the distal phalanx, it is possible to spread the load of the instrument on to the proximal phalanx by either altering the thumb posts on the instrument (see Chapter 13) or providing the musician with a thermoplastic splint contoured to allow playing to continue. For those musicians who develop a painful CMC joint due to excessive

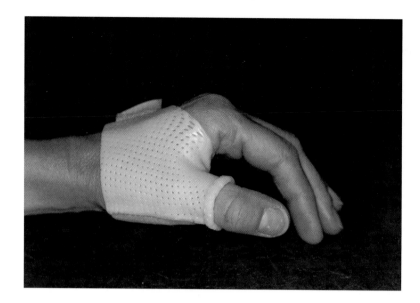

Figure 6

Gauntlet splint to ease loading on CMC joint but allowing functional positioning of the hand and freedom of IP movement.

pinch, we have found that a small gauntlet splint which keeps the thumb in the functional position and prevents excessive adduction while allowing flexion at the IP joint will usually help to alleviate symptoms (Fig. 6). For this type of thermoplastic splint, we use a plastic material which has some drape, but will not stretch uncontrollably. It may be necessary to build up the bow so that the thumb and index finger do not meet to pinch, or indeed on occasion the musician needs to switch from the French to the German style of bow (see Chapter 13). Functional splinting can be used to provide protection of any joint. The exact requirements of splinting must be carefully analysed and the splints must be custom-made to provide an exact fit and to provide the finger position required.

Muscle strengthening and exercise

Joint mobility is a prerequisite for function and must be maintained at all cost. When reduced, joint range must be increased to the degree required for correct technical performance. Passive and active exercises are used from an early point. Prolonged rest and non-playing, in general, must be avoided. Muscle strength and stamina must also be restored to playing requirements following injury. When joint movement is reduced, isometric contraction will help maintain muscle function. Isotonic muscle work, especially against graded resistance, will improve muscle bulk and strength. Therapeutic putty provides a very effective form of exercise, increasing power grip and mobility. Care must be given to the use of dynamic grip exercisers as it has been found that there is an increased incidence of trigger fingers following their usage in the unconditioned young musician, due presumably to direct pressure over the proximal flexor tendon sheaths while active gripping is being performed (Personal communication, U. Büchler). The strengthening of the intrinsic muscles is of vital importance for many musicians, especially those with hypermobility. These small muscles tire easily and quickly, so frequent short exercise sessions are encouraged and are effective. Proprioceptive neuromuscular facilitation (PNF) techniques help facilitate and re-educate muscle contraction/relaxation and co-ordination and encourage normal movement patterns and function.

Sensory re-education

Complete sensory loss in critical tactile areas is not compatible with the effective playing of a musical instrument. Even sensory loss in less critical areas will unbalance playing. However, when sensation is lost or is temporarily lost pending recovery of a nerve, with training additional sensory input can compensate and effective sensibility be achieved. The techniques of sensory re-education are well documented (Wynn Parry 1982) and are well worthwhile for the musician recovering from a nerve injury.

Tired, painful arms and hands

Many musicians' problems seen are due to misuse by constant static loading of muscles usually otherwise employed. This is often seen during extended practice or performance playing without any specific injury (and is characterized by painful, aching, tired muscles). Careful assessment is paramount to ascertain which anatomical structures are involved before a treatment programme is commenced. Contributing factors may include poor posture, poor technique, problems at musician/instrument interface, changes in the musical repertoire, sudden intensification of practice or playing or alteration in practice habit, instrument or chair.

Treatment consists of periods of reduced activity or possibly a short period of complete rest followed by controlled graded exercises and a rigid practice programme. Specific modalities to decrease muscle pain may be required and a re-education programme to prevent further injury or new injury from occurring is essential. Any contributing factors are corrected or modified. The muscles involved may have developed trigger points which prevent them from fully lengthening during the relaxation phase of muscle activity leading to a constant low-grade loading and subsequent pain (Travel and Simons 1983). Specific pain patterns have been recorded. In general terms, trigger points are treated with pressure applied directly on the trigger point until local or referred pain has eased. This may take many minutes and often muscle twitching is felt. Following the easing of pain, a heat pack is applied to the muscle belly and then the involved muscle is slowly stretched to the limit of pain-

free range. The patient is also taught home stretches, which he performs twice daily, having first warmed the muscle.

Acupuncture can also help to alleviate symptomatic trigger points. On occasion muscles have become so accustomed to a shortened contracted position they are unable to relax and elongate to resting length. Cold spray and stretch techniques are most beneficial in this instance. Once again the patient is taught specific home stretches. In addition, examination of the musician's technique should be conducted and alteration made where appropriate. In all instances an overall home care conditioning programme is essential to help prevent reinjury or new injury. General warm-up hand and arm exercises are taught (Leader 1997) and also whole body warm-up and stretching, especially for the upper limbs. Practice schedules should be well-structured and practising should not extend beyond 20 minutes and should be interspersed with rest periods during which general mobility exercises, stretching and relaxation should be carried out. General body fitness is important and participation in non-contact and non-ball contact sports is to be encouraged. Body awareness is also important and great benefit can be gained from yoga, or the Alexander and Feldenkreis techniques.

Hypermobility

Hypermobility (see Chapter 7) or excessive joint laxity can be a cause for non-specific diffuse aches and pains in the musician's hand. It can often go undiagnosed for many years, but once it has been diagnosed great benefit can be obtained from a specific exercise programme. Due to the joint instability from abnormally lax ligaments, muscles supporting the joint compensate by increasing their normal muscle effort in an attempt to stabilize the joint. If this increase in muscle effort fails to stabilize the joint, further stretching, together with associated tendonitis, joint sprain and laxity occurs. This increase in muscle load leads to discomfort in the muscle bellies after only short periods of playing and can in severe cases inhibit playing altogether. The small muscles of the hand, the intrinsics and lumbricals, and antagonistic muscle groups, wrist extensors and flexors, are often involved.

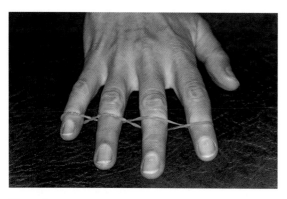

Figure 7

Strengthening exercises for the intrinsic muscles of the hand against the resistance of a rubber band.

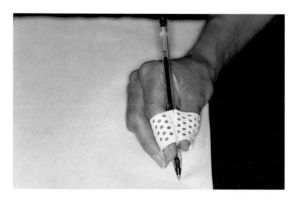

Figure 8

A small writing-aid splint especially useful for the young hypermobile patient required to write for extended periods 'sparing' joints for musical practice and playing.

Hypermobility is more common in females than males and often has a peak incidence in the mid-teens, often when there is great demand on the youngster's hand from increased writing in preparation for examinations or intensive playing to achieve greater success in music competitions and examinations. Once diagnosed, careful assessment and treatment with a hand therapist is essential. It is important to ascertain which joints are hypermobile by carefully studying playing posture, especially after a period of playing to see any resulting 'tired' posture. Careful assessment of the muscle power of individual muscles supporting the involved joints is paramount, for the basis of treatment is to strengthen these muscles specifically. Normal therapeutic measures are initially used for any accompanying joint sprains and tendonitis. A very specific exercise programme is then individually tailored to strengthen the muscles controlling the hypermobile joints, usually the intrinsic muscles of the hand and the wrist and finger extensors. Various exercises providing steadily increasing resistance are given – elastic bands, marbles for finger football, therapeutic putty, pencil and beer mat flicking are a few ideas (Fig. 7). General arm exercises for the large, more proximal muscle groups are also encouraged. The musician must be made aware of the importance of these exercises and the need to persevere. Results do not happen overnight – the smaller intrinsic muscles tire easily. The motto 'little and often' is most important. Musical practice time is limited to pain-free playing several times a day, rather than for longer periods. Posture awareness is also important and necessary correction is attempted. Weight-relieving straps and supports and possible instrument modification may be necessary to decrease the strain on the lax joints. A small writing-aid splint (Fig. 8) can make all the difference to cramps and aches in writing, so alleviating stress and loads with this activity and allowing increased musical practice time. By understanding and carefully following a tailored, specific-muscle-strengthening exercise programme, the musician suffering from hypermobility will slowly gain benefit as the muscles increase in strength and stamina and the joints are increasingly supported.

Acute injury, strains and sprains (excluding the PIP joint)

Acute injuries in the musician rarely occur from instrumental playing. They are usually the result of unaccustomed sporting or DIY (home improvements) activities often leading to tendonitis and synovitis. Immediate treatment consists of complete rest for 48 hours, ice, elevation and non-steroidal anti-inflammatory preparations.

Ultrasound can be most useful to speed up the resolution of the inflammatory process. Protective splinting to rest the part may also be indicated. Following 48 hours of complete rest, gentle graded exercises are introduced, together with protected practising for 5 minutes, twice daily. This is increased in increments at 3- to 4-day intervals, as indicated by continuing absence of pain. Home care guidelines are discussed and implemented. It is of note that this is one of the few instances when a complete cessation of playing may be beneficial, but this period should be minimized, ideally to no longer than 48–72 hours.

Acute injury of the PIP joint

Injuries around the PIP joint are some of the commonest and the most difficult to treat in musicians. These injuries tax the skill and patience of the most dedicated. They require utilization of virtually every technique and appliance in varying sequences and also require judgement by the therapist in finding the correct ratio between exercise and rest to regain motion while not reinjuring the joint. In the musician occasionally one has to compromise range of movement in one direction to secure extra range in the other functional playing direction.

The PIP joint is intolerant of injury, which usually has been sustained in some non-musical activity. It may be a direct injury to the joint (fracture, dislocation, ligament avulsion or sprain) or to the periarticular structures, particularly the extensor tendon mechanism (closed rupture, avulsion or laceration). With all of these injuries the joint swells, falls naturally into position of 20–30° of flexion and places the extensor mechanism on stretch. Contracture of the joint rapidly develops (in 5–10 days) and the extensor mechanism attenuates, allowing the central part to elongate and the lateral elements to slide volarly beyond the axis of the joint, creating additional flexion deformity of the PIP joint and hyperextension of the distal interphalangeal joint (DIP) – the boutonnière deformity. The hand therapy of these injuries focuses on:

- Prevention of the deformity
- Maintenance of full extension of the PIP joint while inflammation settles and healing

progresses, while also maintaining mobility at the DIP joint
- Recovery of motion (flexion) while preventing the deformity from recurring.

The treatment naturally falls into three phases, although in any one situation the phases may overlap.

Phase I

In the acute phase before contracture has developed, the finger must be maintained in full extension using a static splint for 7–10 days until inflammation and swelling have settled. If early contracture has developed this must be overcome using steady stretching via a dynamic splint. When full extension has been obtained, the joint must again be rested for 7–10 days in full extension. Occasionally surgical release may be required before full extension can be obtained. The postoperative regime is identical from that point onwards.

Phase II

Chronic swelling can be controlled by Coban wrap and massage, and mobilization is started, protected by a dynamic splint or using intermittent active flexion exercises and a removable static extension splint. The extension splint must be worn at night. Short practice sessions on the instrument are started at this time if technically possible. The DIP joint must be kept fully mobile (Fig. 9).

Phase III

This is the phase of recovery of functional motion, and can be started whenever phase II has been initiated and there has been no recurrence of effusion in the joint or of the flexion deformity. If the musician requires full extension, very little change is made from the regime of phase II except that the patient is weaned off protective splinting and controlled active flexion is allowed. If the musician requires full flexion at the PIP and DIP joints (the DIP should be fully mobile at this point as it has been deliberately

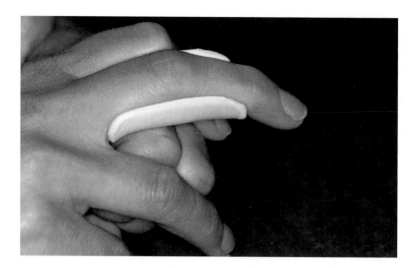

Figure 9

Removable static PIP splint, allowing full mobility of the DIP joint
which is essential in phase II of
rehabilitation of PIP injuries.

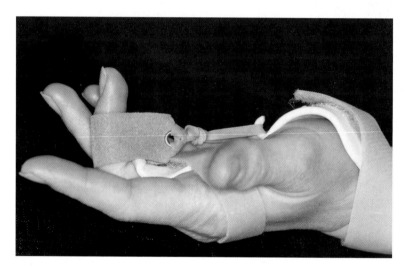

Figure 10

Custom-made dynamic splint useful for regaining PIP flexion in
musicians who require extreme
flexion. Some extension lag may
develop and may have to be
accepted.

mobilized throughout phase II), passive stretching either manually or by dynamic splinting by
rigid custom-made thermoplastic splint manufactured specifically for this task (Fig. 10) is added
to the regime. This is the situation with most
violin and viola players who require 50–60° DIP
flexion and 90°+ of PIP flexion. To obtain this
amount of flexion following injury to the PIP joint
or adjacent extensor mechanisms requires rigorous dynamic flexion devices during phase III, and
almost certainly 5–10° of full active extension
may be lost. However, passive full extension
must be maintained during this period by static

extension splinting used alternately with dynamic
flexion, splinting and exercise. Conversely, some
woodwind players play in a mild boutonnière
position (Fig. 11) and indeed a degree of the original deformity may need to be created in phase III
at the expense of flexion before the instrumentalist can comfortably return to the clarinet or
oboe!

The musician patient has to be alerted at the
outset to the complexities of this type of injury,
which may have seemed trivial at the time. The
musician must also be alerted to the timeframes
and temporary disruption of playing schedules

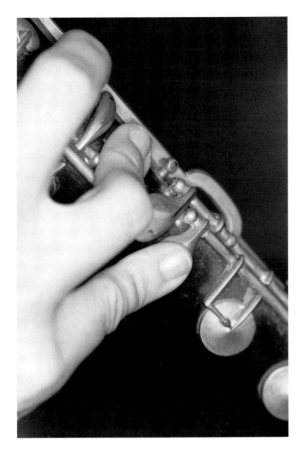

Figure 11

Mild boutonnière position adopted by some woodwind players. Overcorrection of a traumatic boutonnière deformity may have to be slightly 'undone' in this group of musicians.

which may ensue over a 2- to 3-month period. Usually, however, musicians prove to be the ideal patients, being conscientious to the point of obsession with complex regimes. In our experience all have been able to return to full-time playing.

Postoperative care in musicians: Dupuytren's contracture

Dupuytren's contracture release is one of the more common operations performed on musicians (see Chapter 8), and the postoperative hand therapy is critical. The preoperative deformity may vary from a mild digital flexion deformity but with significant loss of span (important in pianists) to a much more severely contracted or recurrently contracted finger with dense scarring which also requires skin-grafting. In our hand therapy department we use a rigid postoperative regime in all cases of Dupuytren's release surgery, modified for the musician.

If the surgery does not involve skin-grafting, the patient is kept in a mildly compressive bandage with a plaster-of-Paris splint to maintain extension of the operated digit for 5 days. The hand is kept meticulously elevated at all times and free joints are kept mobile. On the fifth day the dressing is removed and scar management is commenced with a custom-made thermoplastic splint to maintain extension. This is worn day and night for 1 week, being removed only for washing, exercises and limited playing of the instrument. The playing consists of 5-minute sessions two to three times a day, preceded by washing of the hand in warm water to increase mobility. Active and passive flexion and extension exercises are also performed initially under supervision but mostly unsupervised at home. The patient is given instructions on a very specific regime, concentrating on aspects which are critical to his playing and frequently include hyperextension of the digit at the MP joint and wide active abduction of all digits. Advice on wound care is also given and the musician is encouraged to wash his hands frequently under running lukewarm water as an aid to wound toilet and to increase flexibility prior to exercise sessions or playing. A mixer tap facilitates this as it is unsatisfactory to have the patient dangle his hand, dependent and swollen, in a bowl of unclean water.

On the twelfth day the sutures are removed, scar massage is started, a pressure insert may be applied to the splint to apply direct pressure to the early immature scar and the thermoplastic splint can be remodelled and adjusted to encourage further extension. At this point the musician will have been practising on his instrument, albeit for brief periods, and he will be able to discuss specific difficulties that he is experiencing or is anticipating with increasing playing. He can discuss this with the hand therapist and splint adjustment can be made. Little finger

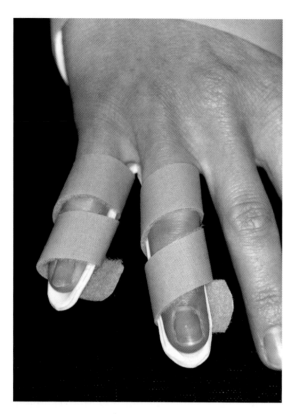

Figure 12

Static extension splint used for postoperative care following release of Dupuytren's contracture. In this case, two fingers have been released and the musician, a pianist, requires wide span. The little/ring finger web will be incrementally widened.

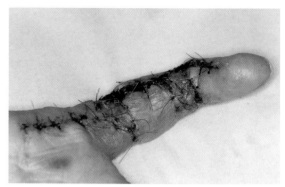

Figure 13

Early skin grafts 5 days after release of recurrent Dupuytren's contracture by local flaps and interposed grafts.

abduction is often a difficulty, so splint adjustment may actually include widening of the span on the splint between the little and ring fingers (Fig. 12) or insertion of an abduction block to the base of the web.

From this point on, the splint is only worn at night for a minimum of 6–8 weeks, but occasionally for 3–6 months if active scarring persists at the operative site. If specific finger abduction is required, the musician may need to use the splint for some hours during the day. Light activities of daily living are encouraged, as well as incremental increase in playing and in the best case full rehearsal level can be achieved by 2½–4 weeks. A full range of finger flexion

and extension will normally have been achieved 4 weeks after surgery. Most musicians have managed to return to performance playing in 6–8 weeks.

If skin-grafting has been necessary, then the exercise part of the regime is delayed 1 week, to allow additional consolidation of the graft. We advise the musician to rest the hand until day 12, only performing very gentle flexion to allow healing of the grafts. A thermoplastic splint, however, is still made on the fifth postoperative day, but it will often be made of perforated material to allow airflow to the wound (Figs 13 and 14). The wound will normally need a light non-stick dressing under the splint. When the wound is well healed, a new splint is made with a more rigid, non-perforated thermoplastic material which is more easily removable. Washing of the wound following skin-grafting is very important and we advise musicians to bathe their hands under running water from the twelfth day to wash away any loose crusts and debris from the edges of the graft site. Exercising under running water is also comfortable and beneficial. Our patients have reported that this makes active movement much easier.

In both non-grafted and grafted cases, light strengthening exercises progressing to heavier resistance are introduced when oedema is controlled and the patient can tolerate pressure to the affected area. Varying grades of exercise

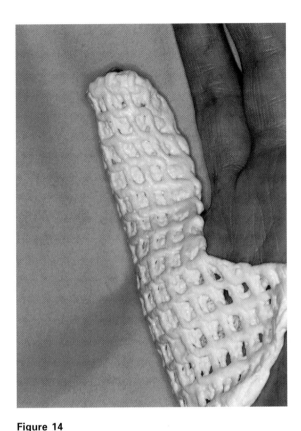

Figure 14

Perforated thermoplastic static extension splint used during early postoperative period on the same case as Fig. 13.

contract into flexion when the splint is left off for the first overnight trial, the musician must watch the affected digit closely over the next few days. If it shows a tendency to contract even after 48–72 hours, then the splint will need to be worn again at least every second night. This process of weaning and monitoring must continue until there is no tendency for further scar contracture to develop. Individuals vary. In our experience, all patients require night splintage for a minimum of 6–8 weeks, but those with a strong propensity to form scar and hypertrophic scar may require splintage for 4–6 months. To date, all professional musicians who have had surgical release of Dupuytren's contracture, with or without skin-grafting, have returned to full-time professional playing. Our experience has demonstrated musicians to be extremely good patients, complying to the letter with the very strict exercise and splintage regimes.

Carpal tunnel decompression

Following surgical decompression of the carpal tunnel, the hand is placed in a bulky, mildly compressive dressing, incorporating a small plaster of Paris (POP) splint on the flexor aspect holding the wrist in 20° of extension. This is felt to be important, as it prevents the unusual, yet potentially devastating complication in the musician of dislocation of the flexor tendons. The surgical dressing is removed between the fifth and the seventh day and the patient is placed in a removable wrist splint, again with the wrist held in slight extension. The importance of wrist splintage at this stage has recently been stressed from personal experience by Goldner (1997). The patient remains in this for an additional 7 days. However, the splint can be removed for the purposes of bathing, and for gentle unresisted wrist exercises and for light finger exercises on the instrument. However, the patient is encouraged, with the splint in place, compulsively to maintain full digital flexion and extension. The stitches are removed between the twelfth and the fourteenth postoperative day and the musician is encouraged to begin graded music strengthening practice at from 10 to 14 days. Most patients are back to full rehearsal level 4 weeks following surgery.

putty are supplied to this effect. Standard measurements are taken throughout the postoperative regime to allow the therapist to monitor progress and to provide the musician with goals and encouragement. The patients are reviewed weekly until they have regained a full range of motion and are playing to a reasonable degree. Once this point has been reached and we are sure that the splint will need no further adjustment, the follow-up visits are more widely spaced. Generally speaking, once musicians have returned to performing, they will no longer need to be seen for routine follow-up. However, the necessity for intermittent splintage for 2–6 months has to be explained and reinforced. If the affected digit does not show a tendency to

Ganglionectomy and benign tumour removal

The surgical removal of ganglions is relatively more frequent in musicians than in the general population, since the minimal symptoms which these lesions frequently cause are often sufficient to distract a musician or to disrupt or unbalance playing. The postoperative care of musicians having had flexor sheath ganglions removed is simply that of wound care, provided the musician moves the afflicted digits through a complete range of motion within 24 hours of surgery. If there is any suggestion of reluctance on the musician's part to perform this simple task (and this is unusual), then closely supervised active mobilizing regimes have to be utilized within 48–72 hours of surgery.

The postoperative care of musicians having undergone excision of dorsal wrist ganglions is very similar to that described for patients undergoing carpal tunnel release. The initial dressing is mildly compressive and contains a POP splint holding the wrist in slight extension. This is changed to a removable wrist splint on the fifth to the seventh day, but the wrist is maintained in slight extension for at least another week, the splint only being removed for bathing. By the fourteenth postoperative day active wrist flexion has started but the splint is still used as external support when heavy lifting or gripping is required. Scar massage is also utilized at this time and the patient continues this for 3–4 months. If good wrist mobility has not been achieved 4 weeks from surgery, passive stretching of the wrist is started. Although significant residual wrist stiffness can be expected for at least 8 weeks, permanent loss of mobility is unusual. There is commonly some loss of co-ordination following surgery and the normal fluid playing of the instrument takes some time to return, especially if a high level of activity is involved. Therefore ganglionectomy may be disruptive to a musician's playing schedule for longer than anticipated and this must be planned in. This is particularly so in instruments in which wrist flexion is important. The converse, however, is also true – that in instruments in which the playing position requires only wrist extension (cf. woodwinds) disruption need only be for a very short period.

Tendon injuries

Standard regimes are followed following tendon repairs – controlled active early mobilization with as early a return to the instrument as is practical. It is essential to maintain tendon gliding, especially of the flexor tendons, but dynamic extensor splinting can be used in musicians to minimize the chance of rupture, attenuation and adhesion formation following the repair of extensor tendons. The therapist must also be aware of the exact combined posture of the finger for the successful playing of that particular instrument, and in some cases should be prepared to compromise on active movement in one plane or in one direction to gain additional movement in another when this movement is required for playing.

Fractures

The role of the therapist in the management of fractures in musicians is twofold:

- To provide precision external supporting splints when necessary
- To ensure that all joints proximal and distal to the fracture are fully mobile and functional at the point when the fracture is healed and when the musician is ready to return to playing.

A common source of musculoskeletal pain following injury in musicians is unrecognized residual stiffness in undamaged but associated joints following fracture. The standard techniques of joint mobilization are used and they may be facilitated by the use of precision custom-moulded thermoplastic splints providing support to the fracture but sparing adjacent joints.

Neck and shoulders

Jane Kember

A musician presenting with a hand, wrist or forearm problem poses a diagnostic challenge.

Are there local structures responsible or is this a referred pattern? For example, symptoms could result from direct injury to the wrist or originate in a more proximal joint, such as the shoulder, which is referring symptoms to the elbow and forearm. Frequently the spine is the culprit in a distal problem (Maitland 1986a).

An appropriate physical examination is then carried out. By analysing the history, symptom presentation and behaviour, a rational decision on the treatment can be made.

History

Good history-taking is essential. It should cover onset, possible trauma (recent or past) and general medical health. The presentation of the pattern of symptoms and their behaviour under aggravating and easing factors all give clues to the pathology involved (Maitland 1986b). These are tested through range or to the start of pain. Overpressure at the end of range is applied, if painfree. Questions should be focused on changes in technique, instrument, teacher and workload. Competent treatment is only possible if a thorough physical examination of the whole upper body is performed, with observation of spinal and pelvic symmetry linked to the posture in weightbearing.

Objective examination technique

The examination includes:

1. Observation of posture in sitting, standing and playing (undressed)
2. Physical examination of the joints, muscles and soft tissues.

Static muscle tests help to pinpoint muscle or tendon involvement. Changing response may be due to pain or neurological involvement.

Skeletal observation

Observe the posture of the standing patient from the front, the back and from the side. Changes in the spinal curves may be present in all planes; viewed from the back there may be scoliosis, or from the side, an increased kyphosis. The patient is at this time in static posture and this position should be noted for it is a baseline from which to work and is the position that the patient will return to after movement. Viewing from the back, check to see if the shoulders are level and if the angle of the head is normal. Is the head tilted slightly or rotated to one side? Observe the position of the arms. Is there an increased internal or external rotation of the upper arm? If present, a subsequent overcorrection of pronation or supination may follow in the forearm. The posture of the hand in the relaxed position, hanging by the side, will confirm a muscle imbalance. The hand should rest with the palm facing the body, not backwards or forwards. Are the scapulae set high, wide from the spine and rotated? This will alter the subsequent positioning of the arm and hand.

Viewing from the side, observe the head-on-neck, neck-on-shoulder posture. This is one of the most important areas in which pathology may occur, giving rise to distal symptoms. The 'poking chin' posture, with an increased cervical lordosis, upward tilt of the chin and increased extension of the occiput on C1, shifts the whole head forward on the cervicothoracic junction. If a visual 'plumb line' is drawn from the ear to the shoulder, the ear should be directly above the acromion. Frequently the ear is well forward of the shoulder. Soft tissues can be stressed in this abnormal posture and may produce symptoms either at rest or when an activity is attempted. A lateral view also gives a good angle to observe the shoulder posture and any kyphosis in the thoracic spine. The scapula should be flat on the ribcage maintaining the humerus directly below the ear. Muscle imbalance around the shoulder girdle alters the hanging position of the arm, usually into a more forward posture, and changes the dynamics of the whole arm. All this information can be gleaned before touching or moving the patient.

Physical examination

The irritability and severity of the condition having been assessed by history, a physical examination of the movements of the joints and soft tissues is performed. This provides information about pain, restriction and ease of movement. Even if movement appears to be full and free, one should ask the patient if there is any 'pull or block' felt at the limits. This could be significant if hunting for a slight or subtle abnormality. The joints and tissues which need to be examined are those which lie directly under the area and any potential sources of referred pain. Many of the forearm and hand problems presenting for treatment have a direct causal link with cervical and thoracic spine posture and muscle imbalance around the sequela.

Neurological examination

If there are any neurological symptoms, such as paraesthesias numbness or muscle weakness, further checks on sensation to light touch, reaction to temperature and reflexes are performed. Any odd feelings of heaviness of the limb, colour changes or swelling of the hands are noted as they may be linked with the autonomic system. Neural tension tests are performed to check neural mobility (Butler 1991). The free gliding of the nerve through the tissues may be restricted by joint or muscle inflammation, local scar from old trauma or entrapment at one of the known tight spots. A patient presenting with a condition which is highly irritable and who is in severe pain will, of necessity, have a reduced examination, i.e. no end-of-range joint movements or resisted muscle testing. Those patients with chronic symptoms will need more searching tests and observations of subtle changes in joint range, movement patterns and neural tension tests.

Much can be gained from the initial observation of the upper part of the body, unclothed, before movement testing or palpation of soft tissues. Many patients will think that this is odd as they have 'only come for their finger'. One needs to explain about possible causes of symptoms arising in the neck and shoulder. When making the first appointment, the musician is requested to bring the instrument so that playing posture may be observed. The head and neck position may alter during action and the sitting or standing pelvic stance often changes to imbalanced weightbearing, altering the lumbar and thoracic spine curves. It is useful to have access to a piano and the drummers can bring a practice pad to demonstrate techniques. Every instrument has its own problems, as may be seen from previous chapters, and a knowledge of these difficulties can help to

decide if this is a person who needs physiotherapy or specialist instrumental technical advice. The presenting symptoms may be *caused* by playing or may be a condition which could affect anyone but this person *happens* to be a musician.

Treatment

A treatment plan should be drawn up on the basis of findings from the initial examination. This may be adjusted as treatment progresses and presenting symptoms change or diminish. Aims for a typical pattern of treatment are listed here but it must be stressed that this is not a 'recipe' and each case should be treated individually. The order of treatment depends on the irritability of the tissues, joint dysfunction and muscle imbalance and does not follow any set routine. The stabilization of the head, neck and trunk are of key importance in the use of the limbs. Spinal dysfunction is frequently associated with faulty alignment, poor stabilization and abnormal movement patterns. It follows that limb function is altered if the core stability of the trunk is faulty. The patient in Figures 15, 16 and 19, will be used as an example of the following aims and methods of treatment.

Aims

1. To improve the head-on-neck and the neck-on-shoulder posture by mobilizing the cervical spine, stabilizing and strengthening the appropriate muscles and re-educating the proprioceptive feedback to enable an improved posture to be maintained.
2. To mobilize and strengthen joints and muscles of the thoracic spine, reducing the slight kyphosis.
3. To address the muscle imbalance around the shoulder girdle in order to improve the position of the scapula on the thorax and to decrease the forward holding of the glenohumeral joint.
4. To re-educate the pelvic and trunk posture in standing and sitting, with and without the instrument.
5. To mobilize, strengthen and re-educate forearm, wrist and hand function. This has been discussed in the previous section.

Method

1. To improve the head-on-neck and the neck-on-shoulder posture. Movement range is tested actively, passively and with overpressure, as necessary, indicating the level of joint dysfunction: any loss of motion, resistance or pain. Palpation of the individual joints confirms these findings; typically, there is limitation of range in the occiput C1 joint which is a key factor in the 'nodding' or high upper cervical flexion movement. At this level, the muscles act primarily as stabilizers of the head on the cervical spine. The suboccipital extensors, in the absence of appropriate deep anterior stabilization, can become over-tight and contribute to excessive upper cervical extension mobility and poor holding posture. Tightness may not be the primary dysfunction so the muscle pattern must be carefully analysed. The high cervical joints are mobilized, and this, combined with re-education of the upper cervical stabilizers, in lying and sitting, is part of the process of posture retraining. Tight scaleni and sternocleidomastoids may need gentle stretching. The general rule is to *stabilize* before strengthening and attempt to *shorten* the lengthened muscles inducing a reciprocal relaxation and lengthening of the tightened muscles. If there is a long-standing tightness, gentle stretch techniques are used for specific muscle groups. A programme of exercises to improve neck movements, especially head retraction and high cervical flexion, is given. These should be done slowly and, if possible, in front of a mirror.

The patient must understand that regular, specific exercise, over a long period, is an important adjunct to the mobilizations and muscle work done in the session. It is very important to follow up the work done after therapy with appropriate continual posture awareness and exercises. The responsibility for recovery is a shared experience and no one should expect to be 'made better' without any effort made by themselves.

2. To mobilize and strengthen joints and muscles of the thoracic spine. The thoracic spine needs to be mobile and held in a good posture to allow the head and arms to function well. The common tendency, linked with the poking chin posture, is an increased kyphosis, with decreased flexibility in the ranges of thoracic extension and rotation. Mobilizations of the spine and associated rib junctions will give greater freedom of movement.

This is especially important in wind players, as a freely moving ribcage is essential for good chest expansion and breath control. A fixed area in the thoracic spine also limits the correct alignment of the scapula, altering the angle of the gleno-humeral joint and movement patterns of the limb.

To start with, simple thoracic exercises are given:

- In sitting, rotations with relaxed, folded arms
- Trunk flexion with relaxed arms down to the feet and a slow careful unravelling of the spine, segment by segment, to increase range and awareness of the spinal movement
- Side flexion in sitting and standing and thoracic extensions with arms over the back of a chair.

Emphasis is placed on correct pelvic stability during performance of the exercises in order to prevent distorted movement patterns. Progression to more difficult exercises is closely linked with the retraining of any muscle imbalance in the shoulder girdle and pelvis. It is most important to maintain core stability in slow, controlled exercises before increasing speed, leverage or weight.

3. Muscle imbalance. Muscle imbalance around the shoulder girdle is a major cause of symptoms in a musician. Muscle has two main functions of stability and movement. Some muscles have both functions, especially the erector spinae, serratus anterior, infraspinatus and the rhomboids. Imbalanced muscles show either overactivity and tightness or inhibition and thus functional weakness. The imbalance is an integral part of postural defects, with an adaptive response, over time, leading to poor posture. When analysing any fault in the humeroscapular movement pattern, it is important to note the quality of the action as well as range.

Common muscle imbalance problems are:

- An unstable scapula in the first stages of movement. This is shown by early lateral rotation of the inferior angle and posterior lift of the medial border away from the thorax
- A high, fixed, protracted scapula, often linked with impingement syndromes.

In Figs 15 and 16 the scapulae are held high on the thorax and in protraction. The distance from the spine to the medial border of the scapula is

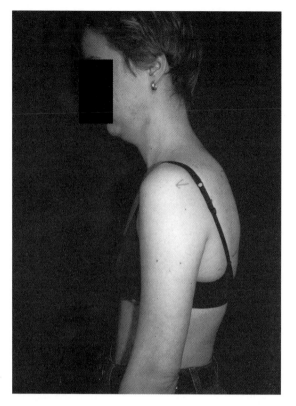

Figure 15

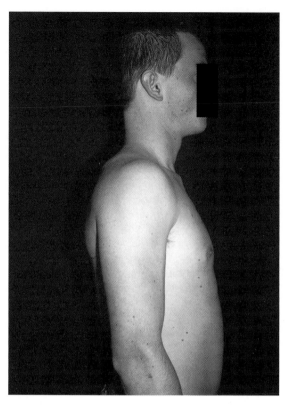

Figure 17

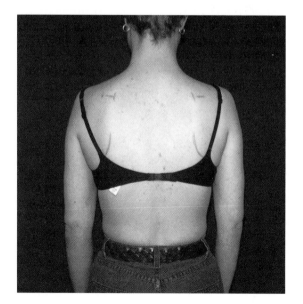

Figure 16

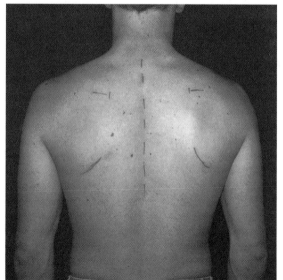

Figure 18

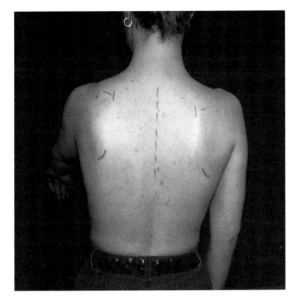

Figure 19

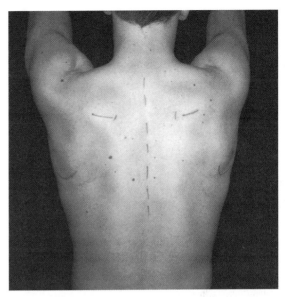

a

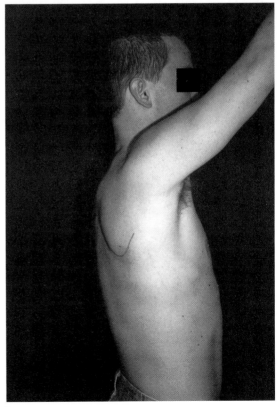

b

Figure 20a, b

excessive, producing an anterior/superior shift of the glenoid cavity. Consequently, the starting position for the glenohumeral movement is altered. Figs 17 and 18 show a better posture of the neck-on-shoulders. A plumb line dropped from the ear should be aligned with the acromion. The scapulae are well spaced and good muscle balance allows correct placement on the thorax.

In Fig. 19 there is an alteration of the humeroscapular rhythm on the left. There is early movement of the inferior angle of the scapula around the thorax at 45° arm elevation. At this range of elevation, there should be a stabilizing pattern, rather than active gliding, to allow arm action. Observe the difference in Fig. 20. The scapulae are held in a good stabilizing posture, flat on the thorax, with both arms in elevation. This is how the shoulder girdle provides a stable base from which the arm can move freely and in a dissociated manner from the scapula.

Retraining of specific muscle groups is undertaken to correct muscle imbalance. Exercises are *low effort* to recruit tonic fibres for stability. Work is performed in the inner range with emphasis on increasing the holding time. The aim is to change the length of the muscle and the motor recruitment. For example, work on the inferior trapezius is taught in lying, prone kneeling and sitting. It is then related to the playing postures. Strengthening should take place only after the imbalance has been addressed. There must be a change of motor recruitment and an alteration of length to weakness or shortness to tightness before attempting any strengthening of the muscles. If this is not achieved, progressive strengthening work will reinforce the incorrect patterns.

There may be a change in upper arm and forearm position associated with the altered scapular posture and movement. Correct humeroscapular movement places the limb in the correct position for the function of the hand. Any alteration in the shoulder girdle posture causes a reciprocal adaptation in the limb. The upper arm may rotate internally with a subsequent pronation in the forearm. Consequently, the hand may be used in increased ulnar deviation, e.g. in violin bowing, producing symptoms in the hand. The pianist may adapt by oversupinating the forearm, putting more stress on the ulnar side of the hand and altering the weight transference to the keys.

These may be minor changes, but long-term misuse alters the proprioceptive patterns of the spine and shoulder girdle, giving rise to problems. It is a 'chicken and egg' situation. Is the poor posture present because of underlying joint dysfunction, neural irritation and muscle inhibition or has a continuous bad postural habit induced stiffness, neural tension and change of muscle function? The therapist has to find an avenue into this self-perpetuating cycle and try to re-educate the mechanics and functions of all structures.

Progress may be slow if there has been a long-standing problem but an improvement may be seen after 4–6 weeks. This must be explained to the patient so that regular practice of the exercises is established. It is helpful to give a 'red dot' programme. Small red dots are stuck in various places to remind the patient about posture correction and exercise. Helpful areas are on the computer, wristwatch, mirror in the bathroom, music stand and any other areas which catch the eye frequently.

4. To re-educate pelvic and trunk posture. Basic, general posture re-education is a key part of the treatment. As can be seen from the methods used above, there is a great overlap. Good cervical posture is only possible if joint function and stability are linked with adequate muscle balance and neural soft-tissue mobility. This applies to the whole of the body. It is pointless improving the upper posture if there is poor pelvic stability and poor general body proprioception. Observing the body stance in standing, sitting and playing demonstrates alterations in weightbearing. Commonly, an upper thoracic kyphosis produces an increased lumbar lordosis, with an anterior tilt of the pelvis. Weight may be taken more on one leg than the other. If the patient is asked to stand on one leg, the balance on one side may be faulty. In sitting, observe the weightbearing on the ischial tuberosities and check if it is equally distributed. Exercises to promote the recognition of correct proprioceptive feedback are given in standing and sitting. Using a mirror enhances the visual perception and enables more rapid postural correction.

These treatment techniques are used in an appropriate order for each person and the ratio of mobilization to muscle rebalancing will vary.

As can be seen, the whole body should be assessed. A seemingly localized hand problem can develop as a direct consequence of an adaptive change in other areas of the body. Alternatively, a clearly defined hand problem can set off a chain reaction of altered mechanics which produce more proximal problems. Careful assessment and analysis will facilitate more accurate treatment with improved outcomes.

References

Butler DS (1991) *Mobilisation of the Nervous System.* Churchill Livingstone: Edinburgh.

Fess and Philips (1987) *Hand Splinting: Principles and Methods* (2nd edn). Mosby: St Louis.

Goldner JL (1997) *American Society for Surgery of the Hand Correspondence Newsletter* 1997–70.

Leader LO (1997) *Total Physical Preparation for Piano Playing.* Denor Press: London.

Maitland GD (1986a) *Vertebral Manipulation.* Butterworth: Kent.

Maitland GD (1986b) *Peripheral Manipulation.* Butterworth-Heinemann: Oxford.

Travel JG, Simons DG (1983) *Myofascial Pain and Dysfunction*, vol. 1. Williams & Wilkins: Baltimore.

Wynn Parry CB (1982) *Rehabilitation of the Hand* (4th edn). Butterworth: London.

12
Unique surgical conditions

Yves Allieu, Kamel Hamitouche, Jean-Luc Roux and Yolande Baeten

Introduction

Even if dystonia is the most frequent functional disorder in musicians, some other rare organic disorders must be excluded during a thorough clinical examination (Allieu 1995; Amadio and Russotti 1990). Among these organic disorders, there are some anomalous connections between the flexor tendons at the forearm level which are responsible for pain after continuous effort as in Linburg–Comstock syndrome. There are also well-known connections between the extensor tendons, the conexus intertendinei, which, however, do not normally interfere with digital independency. Sometimes, these conexus intertendinei are too distal and can subluxate at the metacarpal head level, especially at the little finger. This is characterized by a painful trigger. The extensor tendons can also spontaneously subluxate at the metacarpal head level, most frequently in congenital hypermobility. Finally, at the wrist level hypermobility can provoke a synovial ganglion. Even if it is small and invisible this can be responsible for discomfort after effort.

Flexor tendon anomalies

In the literature reports of anomalies of flexor pollicis longus (FPL) are abundant and many anatomical variations are described, e.g. by Macalister (1872, 1889), Wood (1866, 1868), Carver (1869), Gruber (1875), Walsham (1880), Testut (1884), Le Double (1897) and others in the nineteenth century, and more recently by Kaplan (1953). The most frequent anomaly is the additional tendinous connection between the FPL and flexor digitorum profundus of the index finger (FDP II). Sometimes, there is a connection

between FPL and FDP III, the FDP IV, or even the first lumbrical muscle. This additional tendon can even have a muscle belly which is attached to the muscle belly of the FPL. A common flexor tendon to the thumb and index finger has been found as in apes. A common flexor profundus muscle with five tendons, one for each finger, has also been found as in lemurs. Finally, there can be an anomaly of the tendon sheath of the FPL which encloses the FDP II with some thick adherences.

Linburg–Comstock syndrome

In 1979 Linburg and Comstock described a painful disorder at the distal level of the forearm following effort. This is due to an anomalous connection from the flexor pollicis longus (FPL) to the index finger flexor digitorum profundus (FDP), which obstructs independent flexion of those fingers. On clinical examination the patient is unable actively to flex the distal joint of the thumb without simultaneously flexing the distal joint of the index finger. Each passive restriction of this simultaneous flexion of the index finger provokes pain and cramps proximal to the wrist (Fig. 1).

Lombardi et al (1988) reported on 33 cases followed at the Mayo Clinic between 1979 and 1984. All had clinical findings consistent with Linburg–Comstock syndrome. Twenty-four cases were treated surgically. In 15 cases an anomalous tendon was found and in the remaining 9 cases a synovial anomaly was found. There was an improvement in almost all cases after surgery. Unfortunately, the authors did not state whether any patient was a musician.

Rico Aguado and del Pino Paredes (1987) reported on one case in which they found during

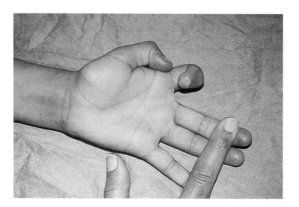

Figure 1

The patient is unable actively to flex the distal joint of the thumb without simultaneously flexing the distal joint of the index finger.

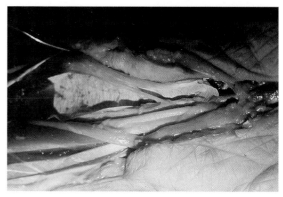

Figure 2

An additional tendon between the FPL and the FDP II was found in five cases.

surgery a common FPL tendon for the thumb and index finger. They split the tendon as far as the musculotendinous junction and this gave better independency of the two fingers.

Takami et al (1996) reported on one case which improved after resection of an anomalous tendon slip. Linburg and Comstock have reviewed 194 patients and found their clinical sign in 89 cases (47%), of which 28 were bilateral. They have also dissected 92 cadaver hands and found in 18 cases an anomalous FPL. In our department we examined 236 individuals and found the clinical signs in 97 cases (36%), of which 24 were bilateral. We also dissected 22 cadaver hands and found an anomaly in 6 cases. In 5 cases we found an additional tendon (Fig. 2) and once we found additional muscle belly with tendon (Fig. 3) (Y Allieu, unpublished work).

The authors have operated on four patients who described pain and discomfort during daily activity of which they did not give the precise nature, and who had a positive clinical result. In all cases the authors found a connection between the tendon of FPL and that of FDP II, consisting of an accessory tendon between the FPL proximally and the FDP II distally. In all cases the excision of this connection gave immediate relief.

As a case report we present a 13-year-old female violinist who had a bilateral Linburg–Comstock sign. This restriction was painful in the left extremity after prolonged rehearsals.* During surgery we found a common FPL (Fig. 4) which we split longitudinally as far as the muscle belly to become a tendon for the thumb and a separated tendon for the index finger (Fig. 5). The independency of the two fingers was partially improved (Fig. 6) and she could play the violin without any complaints.

Other flexor tendon anomalies

Many authors have described anomalies of the flexor digitorum superficialis (FDS), especially at its ulnar border (Wood 1866, 1868; Testut 1884). Apart from the absence of the FDS for the little finger (34% in all individuals according to Baker et al 1981), there also exist anomalous connections between the FDS for the fourth and little finger (18% in normal individuals according to Baker et al 1981). These anomalies are responsible for the loss of independency between these two fingers.

*(Note however that surgery is not always necessary as minor adjustment of technique or changes to the instrument (see Chapter 13) may solve the problem.)

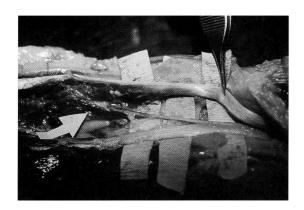

Figure 3

An additional muscle belly with tendon between the FPL and the FDP II was found once.

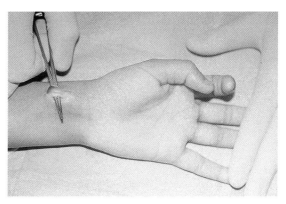

Figure 4

During surgery a common FPL was found to be responsible for the Linburg–Comstock syndrome.

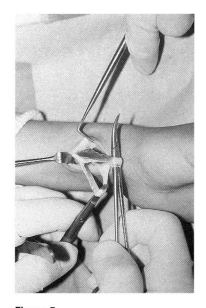

Figure 5

The common FPL was separated longitudinally as far as the muscle belly.

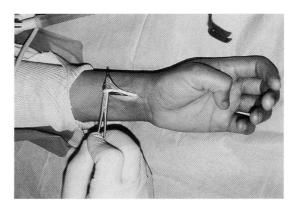

Figure 6

On stretching the FPL the independency of the thumb and index finger was improved.

In 1987 Watson and Kalus reported on a professional guitarist who was restricted during performance due to a lack of independent flexion between the proximal interphalangeal joint of the fourth and little fingers in his left hand. During surgery a connection was found between the FDS for the fourth and the FDS for the little finger at and proximal to the carpal tunnel. This connection was excised resulting in an independent excursion of the little finger. This surgical intervention led to an improvement in the patient's musical performance.

Connections between the FDS and the FDP also appear frequently but are more often than not proximal and therefore do not interfere with function.

Finally, a well-known anatomical anomaly of the lumbrical muscle, consisting of a common lumbrical muscle for two adjacent FDPs, seems to cause no clinical restriction of digital independency.

Anomalies of extensor tendons

The conexus intertendinei or juncturae tendinum

Variations in number and location of the extensor tendons and their connections are frequent and mostly cannot be considered as anomalies. Only the connection by a fascial strip, between the extensor pollicis longus (EPL) and the two extensor tendons of the index finger at the wrist level, has been accepted worldwide as an anomaly and can interfere with the independency of the thumb (Testut 1884).

The existence of the juncturae tendinum between the extensor indicis proprius (EIP) and the extensor digitorum communis (EDC) at the metacarpal level is rare and compromises the independency of the index finger. In 1988 McGregor and Glover (McGregor and Glover 1988) reported the case of a professional pianist in whom they excised with success a connection between the EIP and the EDC III.

The juncturae tendinum between the EDC tendons are almost always constant (Leslie 1954; Kaneff 1963; Schenck 1964; Agee and Guidera M 1980; Brand 1985) and they prevent subluxation of the tendons at the metacarpophalangeal (MCP) joint level. In 1990 Von Schroeder et al classified these juncturae tendinum as type I, II or III. In 1988 Wilhelm observed that lack of flexion/extension independency between two adjacent MCP joints is caused by a tenodesis effect of the deep transverse intermetacarpal ligament.

The juncturae tendinum can compensate for the absence of the extensor tendons. This is often seen at the little finger in which the extensor tendon is replaced by the juncturae tendinum which, coming from the ECD IV tendon, inserts itself in the extensor hood (Schenck 1964).

The juncturae tendinum between the fourth and fifth finger is constant and mostly of type III (Von Schroeder et al 1990). Sometimes it inserts too distally and subluxates at the radial edge of the MCP V joint during flexion of this joint. In 1994 Benatar reported on two cases, one pianist and one flautist. The patients described an annoying trigger during flexion of the MCP V joint. During surgery the above-mentioned anomaly was found and rectified by a proximalization of the junctura tendinum on to the ECD IV.

Non-traumatic intermetacarpal subluxation of the extensor tendon

Spontaneous subluxation of the extensor tendon of one finger is almost always at the ulnar side and occurs suddenly after an unusual effort. It is probably the result of repeated microtrauma which tears the superficial part of the intermetacarpal sagittal band (Ishizuki 1990). In contrast, subluxation of multiple extensor tendons at the MCP level in young patients is a congenital disorder. It almost always involves the third and fourth digit and is sometimes bilateral. It is usually ulnar-sided, but can also be radial. These subluxations are due to the absence of, or a congenital deficiency of, the sagittal bands, or a constitutional hypermobility of the MCP joint which leads to progressive failure of the sagittal bands.

In 1996 Inoue and Tamura reported on four cases of ulnar congenital subluxation in young pianists. This involved the third and fourth digit and was bilateral. The disorder was well tolerated by the non-dominant hand. All cases presented a hypermobility of other joints. All cases were improved after surgical correction using the Elson procedure (1967).

In 1994 Posner and McMahon reported on one case of a 14-year-old (non-musician) patient, who presented a radial congenital subluxation of all the extensor tendons of the long fingers at the MCP level in his dominant left hand. There was also a swan-neck deformity of the long fingers of both hands and an important general hypermobility. The subluxation was improved by surgery at the MCP level, consisting of plication of the radial extensor hood and imbrication of the ulnar extensor hood. The swan-neck deformity disappeared spontaneously after surgery. In our department, we have treated a similar case in a musician by surgical reinforcement of the attenuated extensor hood with an adjacent juncturae tendinum.

Synovial ganglion of the wrist

Constitutional hypermobility can cause a dorsal synovial ganglion of the wrist coming from the scapholunate articulation, especially if the wrist is repeatedly placed in prolonged hyperflexion, such as in pianists and in the left hand of violinists and guitarists. This ganglion can be small and can cause inexplicable discomfort after prolonged effort, the so-called occult ganglion (Berghoff and Amadio 1993; Cardinal et al. 1994). Clinical examination consists of a thorough palpation of the dorsal scapholunate joint with the wrist in different positions. Sometimes ultrasound (Hoglund et al 1994) or MRI (Vo et al 1995) can confirm the diagnosis. Treatment, in our opinion, should be conservative and consists of puncture and infiltration (Finsen 1993), which give good results.

References

Agee JM, Guidera M (1980) The functional significance of the juncturae tendinum in dynamic stabilisation of the metacarpophalangeal joints of the fingers. ASSH proceedings. *J Hand Surg* **5**:288–9.

Allieu Y (1995) Les différents aspects de la pathologie de la main et du membre supérieur des musiciens. *Médecine des Arts* (Numéro Spécial sur La Main du Musicien) **12/13**:3–8.

Amadio PC, Russoti GM (1990) Evaluation and treatment of hand and wrist disorders in musicians. *Hand Clin* **6**:405–16.

Baker DS, Gaul JS Jr, Williams VK, et al (1981) The little finger superficialis – clinical investigation of its anatomic and functional shortcomings. *J Hand Surg* **6**:374–8.

Benatar N (1994) Radial subluxation of the connexus intertendineus at the MP joint of the little finger in musicians treated by connexus intertendineus proximalisation. *J Hand Surg* **18B**:81–7.

Berghoff RA, Amadio PC (1993) Dorsal wrist ganglion – cause of dorsal wrist pain. *Orthopade* **22**:30–5.

Brand PW (1985) *Clinical Mechanics of the Hand*. Mosby: St Louis: 277.

Cardinal E, Buckwalter KA, Braunstein EM, et al (1994) Occult dorsal carpal ganglion – comparison of ultrasound and magnetic resonance imaging. *Radiology* **193**:259–62.

Carver (1869) Irregularities in the arteries and muscles of an idiot. *J Anat Phys* **3**:260.

Elson RA (1967) Dislocation of the extensor tendons of the hand, report of a case. *J Bone Joint Surg* **49B**:324–6.

Finsen V (1993) Aspiration of ganglia in the wrist. *Tidsskr Nor Laegenforen* **113**:950–1.

Gruber W (1875) Ein Fall des Vorkommens des Musculus flexor pollicis longus beim Menschen: als Tensor bursae mucosae tendinum flexorum, oder als Kopf des Musculus digitorum profondus manus. *Archiv Anat, Phys und Wiss Med von Reichert und Du Bois-Reymond* 211–4.

Hoglund M, Tordai P, Muren C (1994) Diagnosis of ganglions in the hand and wrist by sonography. *Acta Radiol* **35**:35–9.

Inoue G, Tamura Y (1996) Dislocation of the extensor tendons over the metacarpophalangeal joints. *J Hand Surg* **21A**:464–9.

Ishizuki M (1990) Traumatic and spontaneous dislocation of extensor tendon of the long finger. *J Hand Surg* **15A**:967–72.

Kaneff DR (1963) Vergleichend-morphologische Undersuchungen über die connexus intertendinei des m.extensor digitorum beim Menschen. *Gegen Morpho Jahrb* **104**:147–78.

Kaplan EB (1953) *Functional and surgical anatomy of the hand*. JB Lippincott: Philadelphia.

Le Double AT (1897) *Traité des Variations Musculaires de l'Homme et leur Signification du Point de Vue Zoologique*. Scheicher: Paris.

Leslie DR (1954) The tendons on the dorsum of the hand. *Aust N Z J Surg* **23**:253–6.

Linburg RM, Comstock BE (1979) Anomalous tendon slips from the flexor pollicis longus to the flexor digitorum profondus. *J Hand Surg* **4**:79–83.

Lombardi RM, Wood MB, Linscheid RL (1988) Symptomatic restrictive thumb–index flexor tenosynovitis; incidence of musculotendinus anomalies and results of treatment. *J Hand Surg* **13A**:325–8.

Macalister A (1872) The mythology of Cheiroptera. *Proc R Soc Lond* **XX**:94–106.

Macalister A (1889) *A Textbook of Human Anatomy: Systemic and Topographical*. Charles Griffin: London.

McGregor I, Glover I (1988) The E-flat hand. *J Hand Surg* **13A**:692–3.

Posner MA, McMahon MS (1994) Congenital radial subluxation of the extensor tendons over the metacarpophalangeal joints: a case report. *J Hand Surg* **19A**:659–62.

Rico Aguado A, del Pino Paredes V (1988) Flexor digitorum profundus common to thumb and index finger, associated with a post-traumatic distal adherence of both tendons. *J Hand Surg* **13B**:72–4.

Schenck RR (1964) Variations of the extensor tendons of the fingers. *J Bone Joint Surg* **64A**:103–10.

Takami H, Takahachi S, Ando M (1996) The Linburg Comstock anomaly: a case report. *J Hand Surg* **21A**:251–2.

Testut L (1884) Muscle long fléchisseur propre du pouce: 469–88; Muscle extenseur commun des doigts and Muscle extenseur propre de l'index: 539–52. In: *Les anomalies musculaires chez l'homme expliquées par l'anatomie comparée, leur importance en anthropologie*. Masson: Paris.

Vo P, Wright T, Hayden F, et al (1995) Evaluating dorsal wrist pain: magnetic resonance imaging diagnosis of occult dorsal wrist ganglion. *J Hand Surg* **20A**:667–70.

Von Schroeder GP, Botte MJ, Gellman H (1990) Anatomy of the juncturae tendinum of the hand. *J Hand Surg* **15A**:595–602.

Walsham (1880) The flexor profundus digitorum inseparably united with the flexor pollicis longus. *St. Bartholomew's Hospital Reports* **16**:85.

Watson HK, Kalus R (1987) Achieving independent finger flexion – the guitarist's advantage. *Med Probl Perform Artists* **2**:58–60.

Wilhelm A (1988) Das Quadriga-phänomen des Strecksehnenapparates und das lig. metacarpeum transversum superficiale. *Handchirurgie Mikrochirurgie Plastische Chirurgie* **20**:173–9.

Wood J (1866) Variations in human myology observed during the session of 1865–1866 at King's College, London. *Proc R Soc Lond* **XV**:235–48.

Wood J (1868) Variations in human myology observed during the session of 1867–1868 at King's College, London. *Proc R Soc Lond* **XVI**:483–524.

13
Adjustment of the musical interface

Robert E Markison

In the course of 35 years of daily music practice and 25 years of professional music-making, I have experienced and self-treated a number of the instrument-specific problems which have become so common among musicians within their long careers. This has resulted in a personal commitment to maintenance of instruments, custom modification of traditional instruments and participation in the development of new musical interfaces. The goals are daily effortless production of music for a lifetime and the care of fellow musicians.

'User-friendliness' and 'user-hostility' have become popular terms for the intuition and comfort that accompany physical interfaces Markison (in press). Human factors engineering seeks to maintain productivity and enhance the pleasure of work and play no matter what the nature of the tools being used. Much of the satisfaction of instrument modification and new design comes from the immediate benefit patients derive from proper changes. Ideas can rapidly be prototyped and implemented without the lag that typically accompanies tool design change for general industry. Limb surgeons are ideally suited to this work because we understand the position of function of the upper limb (Brand 1985). Basic guidelines must derive from the observation of musicians' malfunction: undue forearm pronation and supination are harmful because they stretch fibrous muscle origins and muscle–tendon junctions, shift carpal tunnel contents and place intrinsic and extrinsic muscles at inefficient fiber lengths (Fig. 1). Wrist deviation and extremes of flexion and extension crowd the carpal tunnel and the extensor and flexor compartments. Instruments must be as physically light as possible. Heavy hand-held instruments require weight redistribution through the use of various supports including neck straps, chest harnesses, lap supports and

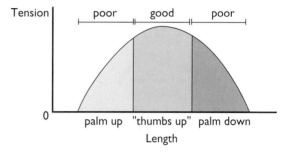

Figure 1

As Paul Brand has clarified in *Clinical Mechanics of the Hand* (1985), muscle fibres work best when they are neither shortened nor lengthened.

posts that go to the player's belt or chair or down to the floor. Poorly maintained instruments cause harm. Adjustability should be built into instruments whenever possible, as anatomy varies significantly from person to person and from hand to hand. Border digits (thumb and little finger) are much abused and should not be given much responsibility in the design of new instruments (Markison 1994).

Computers have given musicians a welcome opportunity to expand their powers in composition, arrangement and performance. Additionally, the computer interface is proving very helpful in training the musical ear and avoiding the pitfalls of single-idiom playing. In other words, by computer interactions with the proper musical instrument digital interface, one can become well versed in the structure of classical and popular music much more rapidly than was possible in traditional pedagogy. All musicians are encouraged to become computer-literate in

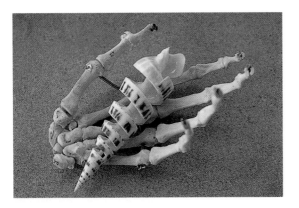

Figure 2

The hand is built upon and moves through the organic spirals of a seashell. Instrument modification and the design of new instruments must respect this wonderful design.

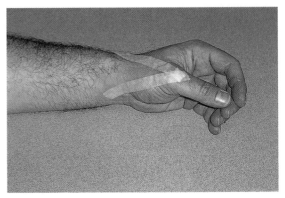

Figure 3

Correct postures can be taught without splinting by the application of tape. Patients quickly modify their behaviours when they learn these taping techniques. The one pictured here preserves the thumb carpometcarpal joint The patient avoids extravagant planes of thumb use because such use will cause the tape to pull and irritate the skin.

order fully to realize their creative powers and develop new income sources.

Being a multi-instrumentalist who is comfortable on wind instruments, string instruments and keyboard instruments, I have learned that it is unnecessarily self-limiting and probably even foolish to play only a single instrument and still expect to be a complete musician.

Many difficulties of the upper limb in musicians flow from failure to use it with respect for its intrinsic design. As we know, the Fibonacci numerical sequence describes the spiral within the sweep of a digit and also describes the spiral of the cross-section of the seashell (Fig. 2). Recalling these natural arcs of design and motion is very helpful as we observe musicians playing their instruments in our clinics. I sometimes apply Micropore surgical tape to help them preserve natural arcs of motion without actually splinting their thumbs, fingers, wrists or elbows. They can learn quickly by their own behavioural modifications when I prevent them from moving through unnatural planes of motion (Fig. 3). The sad fact is that the older and apparently 'primitive' instruments were often more user-friendly than those which we have today (Fig. 4).

In the examples that follow, I will discuss adjustment of conventional musical interfaces

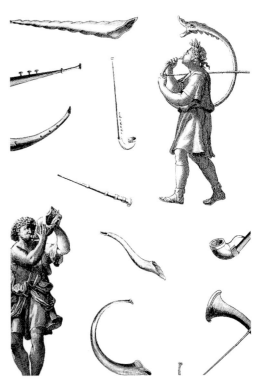

Figure 4

Ancient instruments showed remarkable respect for the organic spirals, as illustrated here.

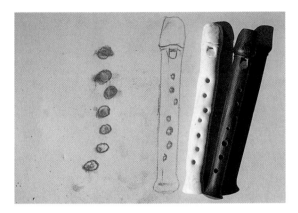

Figure 5

The author begins his recorder fabrication by taking the child's fingerprints, proceeding through sketch and clay prototype to a one-of-a-kind rosewood instrument. The instrument can be played with baroque fingerings or alternative fingerings.

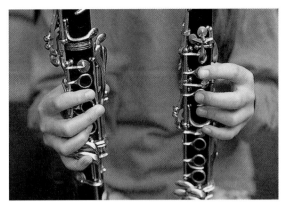

Figure 6

The B-flat clarinet on the left is not appropriate for the hands of young children. The E-flat clarinet on the right is of appropriate scale.

and the value of apparently radical new designs, and I will also offer some considerations about a phenomenum important in healing: improvisational skills.

Designing, making and altering instruments

Fig. 5 illustrates my conception and fabrication of custom-made one-of-a-kind recorders for the small hands of my children. First I had them comfortably place their left index, long and ring fingers and right index, long, ring and little fingers on some paper as they made chalk fingerprints. This provided a comfortable layout for the holes. I drew a quick sketch, then I made a clay prototype so that they could hold it and tell me whether or not they were comfortable. Next, after casting some custom-made tapers, I used a mini-lathe with overhead mill to make recorders out of rosewood. These instruments served beautifully. I taught the children baroque fingering techniques and since I had made some holes larger, I offered them a separate set of alternative fingerings for ease of chromatic scale production and ultimately for greater facility in rapid passage work.

Instrument size and physical weight and relative scale for the musician are important considerations. It would be unwise to expect the average 10-year-old to take up a B-flat clarinet. An E-flat clarinet is ideal (Fig. 6).

In the introductory paragraphs I have described the need to avoid abuse of the border digits, and I have also mentioned the need to avoid sustained wrist flexion. If the bowing technique necessary for playing a cello or double bass is considered, the surgeon immediately becomes aware that the thumb carpometacarpal joint is transmitting a great deal or force and that the wrist rests in the position of Phalen's sign, sometimes leading to median nerve compression. Cellists and double bass players are therefore advised to acquire German bows for practice and/or performance (Fig. 7).

The next generation of violas is very exciting. David Rivinus, an American instrument-designer and fabricator residing in Vermont, has designed the Pellegrina (feminine Italian word for pilgrim). This instrument has a marvellous sound and is truly user-friendly. It has saved the career of Donald Ehrlich, a San Francisco Symphony violist who is pictured playing it here (Fig. 8). Because of the deeper cutaway in the instrument towards the bow hand, the bow angle is more natural. Rivinus has canted the fingerboard

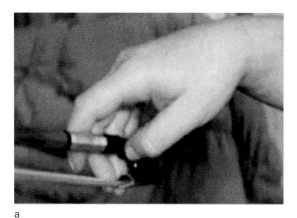

a

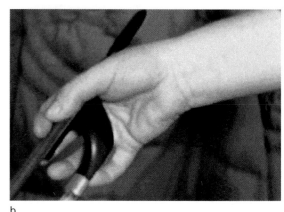

b

Figure 7

The German bow is a helpful tool. (a) Poor thumb and wrist position, (b) Frog is in palm.

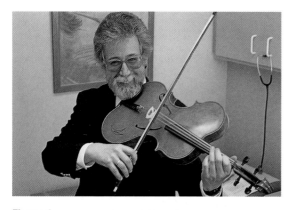

Figure 8

Don Ehrlich, San Francisco Symphony violist, demonstrates the David Rivinus Pellegrina viola. It is an ergonomically sensible instrument with a beautiful tone.

towards the right hand so that the left hand is untwisted. Because of the larger resonance-chambers, the string length is slightly shorter, requiring a shorter cantilever of the left upper limb away from the body. I believe this will permit many string players of the future to break away from the beautiful-sounding but harsh design of the Stradivarius instrument and its many imitators.

As mentioned previously, the golden rule of peripheral muscle fibres is the maintenance of ideal fibre lengths in order to avoid undue shortening and/or stretching and/or twisting that might cause them to fail under repetition or load. (Markison 1990). The left hand of a flautist is unduly twisted and it is best to offer the option of off-axis keys such as those pictured in Fig. 9.

I personally have invented a more radical solution for untwisting the upper limbs of flautists, and the Markison angled flute head joint has an 88° bend which permits untwisting of both upper limbs. A right thumb rest is either soldered on to the instrument or held on by a ring. The left thumb web is kept open by use of a Bo Pep crutch. This head joint has been successfully fabricated by flute-maker Daniel Deitch in San Francisco, California (Fig. 10).

In addition to key repositioning, it is also important to consider the tactile comfort provided by custom-metal-smithed or custom-cast keys. The contrast is obvious here (Fig. 11).

Substitute fingering in wind instruments can be very important for reasons of intonation, comfort, 'navigation' and rapid passage work. Rosario Mazzeo has pioneered many such key extensions which allow right- or left-hand substitute fingers with comfortable fingering combinations (Fig. 12).

Instrument support is nicely provided by struts or posts. Michael Benthin, an American designer,

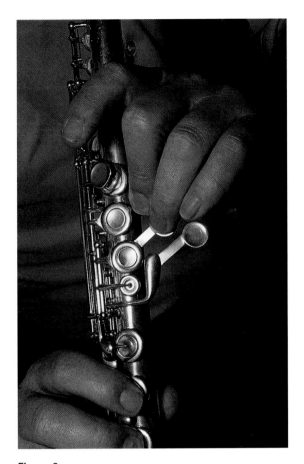

Figure 9

Off-axis key extensions untwist the left hand of the flautist. They also ease the reach of the left little finger, reducing wear and tear for patients who have the 37% prevalent ring–little superficial flexor linkage.

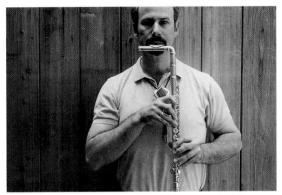

Figure 10

The author has solved his own flute problem by inventing the Markison angled head joint. It provides an 88° bend, a right thumb rest and a spacer for the right thumb web, and sound is not compromised. This has been fabricated by master flute-maker Daniel Deitch in San Francisco, California.

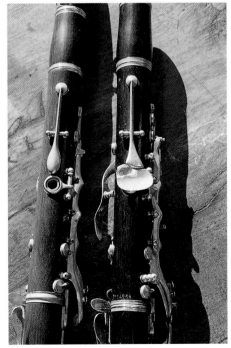

Figure 11

Rosario Mazzeo's custom-built California clarinet, pictured on the left side, redistributes forces very nicely by the custom smithing and casting of silver keys. For some reason, large instrument-makers have not pursued these comfortable modifications.

has developed MUTS, Michael's ultimate thumb-saver. The professional oboist seen here has avoided right thumb carpometacarpal joint reconstruction by using this support, either from a belt attachment or from a seat strap (Fig. 13).

Biofeedback has a valuable role in the modification and design of musical instruments. When EMG leads are applied to the wrist and finger flexors and extensors and to the thumb web muscles, the designer is enabled to work toward least-effort modifications or new designs (Fig. 14).

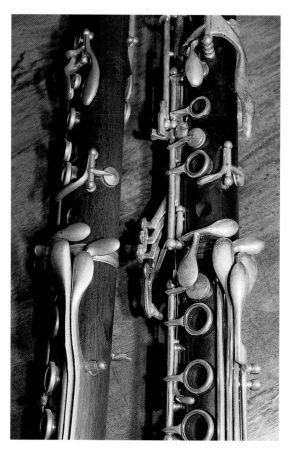

Figure 12

Key extensions and key additions add fingering options for players and also add a great deal of comfort.

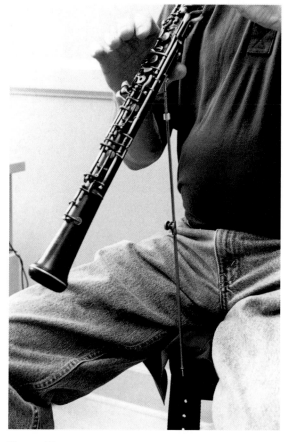

Figure 13

Michael Benthin's MUTS (Michael's ultimate thumb-saver) supports an oboe in this picture. It can just as well support other vertically held wind instruments. The post can come from a belt-melted clip or from a C-strap as in this picture. Supports from the floor can be useful but tend to be more limiting.

Parallel musical interfaces can be very helpful for refining melodic and harmonic ideas. They can also be used independently for performing. Musical instrument digital interface (MIDI) wind instruments such as those produced by Yamaha offer a remarkable range and versatility. They are very lightweight and easy to play (Fig. 15).

I am often surprised at the self-limiting and self-defeating difficulties that befall guitarists. The Dobro and lap steel guitars offer fine opportunities to explore voice-leading, new and different harmonic combinations and some very exciting

ensemble enrichment. The Dobro allows the left hand to hold a steel bar in a relaxed position without undue pronation and the right hand has three or four picks including a thumb pick, again in a position function (Fig. 16).

I have worked with master pedal steel guitarist Maurice Anderson. Anderson is internationally acclaimed for his design effort in the steel guitar and for his complete command of the instrument, including modern jazz recording. He has developed what is called the universal 12-string tuning, and has assisted me in the harmonic set-up of a

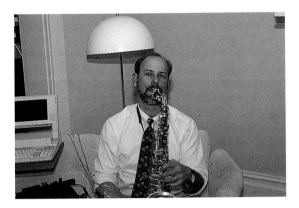

Figure 14

Whenever the author makes changes in instruments, realtime biofeedback electrodes are placed on the communal extensors, superficial flexors, extensor carpi ulnaris, flexor carpi ulnaris and thenar wads. These are integrated through simple software to help keep muscular effort to a minimum throughout the range of the instrument. This is also a nice technique for re-educating musicians' hands.

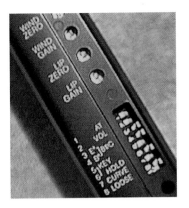

Figure 15

Musical instrument digital interface wind instruments such as the Yamaha WX-7 pictured here offer great opportunities: seven octaves and 128 voices. The author has used this interface to compose and arrange computer-based music.

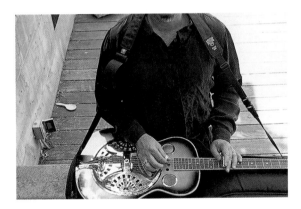

Figure 16

The Dobro seen here is a user-friendly practice and performance alternative to the standard guitar. It does not exclude use of a conventional guitar but it certainly provides better posture with some unique harmonic qualities.

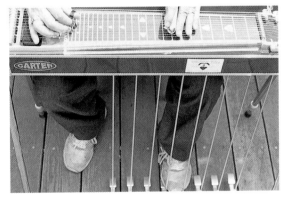

Figure 17

Master pedal steel guitar builder Bud Carter of Carter Steel Guitars has made this pedal steel guitar according to the author's specifications. The string tuning employed has been pioneered by master steel guitarist Maurice Anderson.

pedal steel guitar. The guitar was made by master guitar-builder Bud Carter of Carter Guitars in Mesquite, Texas. By combinations of foot pedal and knee lever usage or application, the 12 strings can be brought through major, minor, dominant, diminished, augmented, extended and very subtly altered chords over a remarkable pitch range. I believe this type of instrument will flourish in the future. I studied privately with Maurice Anderson and quickly realized that the pedal steel guitar is a remarkable composition, arrangement and performance tool (Fig. 17).

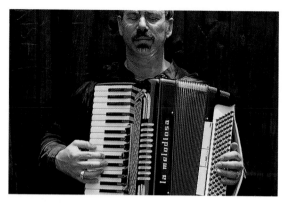

Figure 18

The accordion is a fine instrument which reminds the keyboard player that it is seldom if ever necessary to look at the keys. This avoids a head forward and/or limb forward posture that might transfer undue force to the cervical spine or cause brachial plexus irritation or strain of muscle tendons and nerves distally. Reharmonization is instant and very satisfying on the accordion. The author advises pianists to study the accordion seriously.

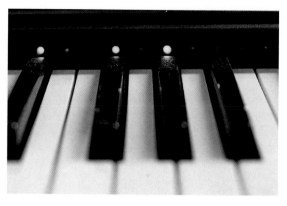

Figure 19

The Yamaha PSR 420 is pictured here. It is unique because lights come on over the keys. Since it is a self-recording instrument, the musician/student can play some chords and phrases, then sit back and listen, preferably learning the 'shapes' of the melodies and harmonies involved. The respite provided by this self-recording, play–listen technique is protective and accelerates learning.

Pianists are mentioned throughout this book. I am surprised to find that few fine pianists have become fine accordionists. The 120 base buttons of the accordion are logically laid out as the root note, a major third above, and then proceeding outward through the major chord, minor chord, dominant chord and diminished chord. The 20 rows of six buttons are arranged in the 'cycle of fifths'. This means that harmonization and reharmonization are instant, simple and infinitely varied using the left hand alone or in combination with the right hand. Since this is a blind melodic, harmonic and rhythmic instrument, pianists are taught that they must 'break away' from looking at the keyboard. I personally have not had great success with those who must watch their hands. Ideally, the pianist will breathe through each musical phrase as though he or she is a wind player, and will not look at the instrument again, just as though playing a wind instrument. I have played the keyboard for a long time and have not found much cause to look at my hands (Fig. 18).

Horizons of music-making

I consider the musical instrument digital interface essential to the development of music-making

and musicianship. I do not personally enjoy the performance of electronic music but I have been successful, as have many others, in the computer-based composition, arrangement, production and sale of music. Income opportunities open for the musicians who have mastered this relatively simple technology.

Electronic keyboards have come down nicely in price, interface easily with computers and have special features including the capacity to store their own data, to transpose materials through various keys and also to act as synthesizers with many voices. The Yamaha PSR 420 keyboard has green lights over the white keys and red lights over the black keys, so a person can watch the key configurations without applying the hands to the keys. In other words, patient-generated or computer-generated melodies, harmonies and rhythms can be studied by 'shapes'. This is a remarkable teaching/learning tool (Fig. 19).

Virtual instruments are coming along nicely, and the best of them have some tactile interaction consisting of ideal postures, minimal force and avoidance of undue repetition. One such successful interface is called 'Thunder', invented and produced by Don Buchla of Berkeley, California.

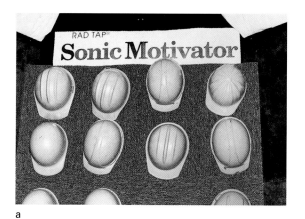
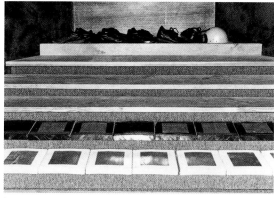

a   b

Figure 20

(a, b) Rosie Radiator, inventor and teacher of the Radical Tap tap dancing technique has invented vibration- and position-sensitive flooring (the Sonic Motivator), which is in itself a unique new musical instrument of many voices, permitting the tap dancer to be a hands-free musician.

In my quest to become a complete musician (Green and Gallwey 1986), I have also studied tap dance, the most musical of dance forms, with a revered California teacher of her own form of tap dance called Radical Tap. Her name is Rosie Radiator. It may seem odd to discuss tap dancing in a chapter about preserving the musician's hand, but I feel that it is entirely appropriate to look also at hands-free music-making. The Radical Tap technique emphasizes avoidance of stress to any body parts. I can confirm this since I have studied with Ms Radiator. Dance teachers from around the world come to her studio to learn how to teach her method. She has invented and pioneered a special musical flooring and circuitry which turns the floor into a musical instrument, and the floor responds to the pressure and position of the tap dancers' shoes for the production of melodies, harmonies and rhythms via instrumental voices selected by the dancer. For example, the dancer can 'play' vibraphones, a full set of drums, a piano, wind instruments, etc. by the action of tap shoes on the special floor panels of this instrument which Ms Radiator calls the Sonic Motivator (Fig. 20). I envisage the use of this device for hands-free music-making, music and dance composition and choreography, music and dance education,

physiotherapy and the development of 'complete artists' who must spare their upper limb for long careers. This is an exciting new instrument.

Finally, I believe that improvisation is the key to musical success. I have noticed over the years that non-improvising musicians suffer far more psychosomatic pain than improvising musicians. The reason is actually quite simple: if they do not improvise, they are consigned to recreating music made by others. Serious classical musicians know that Bach, Mozart, Schubert and Chopin were all ready improvisors. The great jazz pianist Oscar Peterson took a year to study Chopin quite seriously because he knew that Chopin's extended chord structures anticipated modern jazz. I do not ask classically trained musicians to forsake classical music, but the musicians invariably improve the quality of their classical work once they understand the theory and harmony so vital to improvisation. I offer the following list of exciting resources for all musicians.

Resources

1. The best source for all instructional jazz materials including play-along CDs and tapes, books and videos is Jamey Aebersold

Jazz, P.O. Box 1244, New Albany, IN 47151-1244. There are now 70 play-along volumes that include a remarkable number of standard tunes.

2. Mark Levine, a superb bay area pianist and educator, has written two absolutely essential books which should be read and studied by all musicians. The first is *The Jazz Piano Book* (1990) and the second is *The Jazz Theory Book* (1996). Both are published by Chuck Sher Publications, CA.

3. *Jazz Keyboard Voicings and Harmony* by Phil DeGreg, is a wonderful resource. It includes the simplest shell voicings for keyboard and goes out to the most complex Bill Evans types of voicings. A companion set of MIDI files is available.

4. Listening is an absolute must for musicians. The best single source for jazz CDs and at best prices is the 'Double Time Jazz Catalog Discount Jazz Recordings', available from Double Time Jazz, P.O. Box 1244, New Albany, IN 47151.

5. For those who wish to become MIDI-literate, all the current computer platforms support a number of good programs. One of my favourite interactive jazz-oriented programs is Band-In-A-Box Professional, available from PG Music Incorporated, 266 Elmwood Avenue, Unit 111, Buffalo, New York 14222. The same company has two outstanding volumes of superb piano digital files entitled *The Jazz Pianist*, vols I and II. Another favourite interactive jazz-oriented program is called MiBAC Jazz.

6. A lot of musicians fail to warm up. First of all, they should prehydrate by drinking a litre of water before they play. Dry muscles, tendons and nerves do not work very well. Stretches are helpful, and although I have my own set to offer musicians, I advise them to get the videotape entitled 'Therapeutic Exercises for Musicians', nicely done by Richard Norris.

7. There are some after-market extensions to the software named above. Bob Norton, of Norton Music in Florida, has come up with some wonderful accompaniment and chord-progression-type sequences for hundreds of standard tunes, saving the musician the need to program all of these into the computer.

8. Musicians should always 'dialogue back and forth to tape'. This allows them to play back their own materials. The Marantz portable tape recorder permits half-speed playback and also allows very precise pitch tuning. Within the past 6 months Akai has come out with the Riff-o-Matic, which is basically a very small portable digital sampler that samples 13–26 seconds of input and can play it back at half speed or two-thirds speed without any change in pitch. This is done digitally and involves some break-up of sound, but it is a rather remarkable little device. It has been coming into quite a few music stores over the past few months.

9. I have treated many musicians over the past 20 years and I am delighted to receive correspondence from them regularly in appreciation of their new-found improvisational skills. I never suggest that classical musicians forsake their classical music in the name of improvised material, but they all agree that classical music is sweeter and more comprehensible when they have a background in the true theory and harmony of music gained through improvisation.

10. There are ergonomic reasons for keyboardists in particular to study piano voicings. Extravagant reach can always be avoided by proper use of chord inversions, proper voice leading and variation of voicing techniques from the most spare shells to more complex harmonic devices.

11. As stated above, listening is very important. Two of the greatest contributors to the art of jazz in the twentieth century have been Art Tatum and Bill Evans. A regular diet of their music provides lifelong inspiration.

Acknowledgements

Special thanks are due to clarinet teacher Peter Ferrara, clarinet designer Rosario Mazzeo, flute-maker Daniel Deitch, steel guitarist and master musician Maurice Anderson, master steel guitar builder Bud Carter, tap dance instructor and inventor Rosie Radiator, master string-instrument-maker David Rivinus, and many others who have had the courage continually to rethink music-making and musical instrument design.

References

Brand PW, ed. (1985) Mechanics of individual muscles at individual joints. In: *Clinical Mechanics of the Hand*. Mosby: St. Louis: 192–309.

Green B, Gallwey WT (1986) *Inner Game of Music*. Anchor Press: New York.

Markison RE (1990) Treatment of musical hands: redesign of the interface. *Hand Clin* **6**:525–44.

Markison RE (1994) Hands of fire: how to recognize, treat and avoid occupational hazards of keyboard performance. *Keyboard Magazine* April 1994: 93–110.

Markison RE, Johnson AL, Kasdan ML (in press) Comprehensive care of musical hands. In State of the Art Reviews: Occupational Medicine. Hanley & Belfus: Philadelphia.

14
Dystonia

Focal dystonia

Christopher B Wynn Parry

This is one of the most devastating conditions that can affect the musician. It is a form of occupational cramp and is of the same nature as telegraphists' cramp, writers' cramp and other occupational cramp disorders that have been known since the time of Gower's description in the late nineteenth century. It is best described as a painless incoordination of the fingers or, in the case of wind players, the embouchure. Often the musician will describe the finger as being disobedient, refusing to straighten after flexing, being out of control.

The musician begins to realize that he is losing control of his fingers or his lips and that a particular digit or digits are becoming disobedient and will not do what he requires. The classic example is the pianist who finds he cannot stop the ring and little fingers of the right hand curling into his palm, while at the same time the middle finger may extend. A guitarist may find that he cannot control the right middle finger and the cellist finds that the right thumb will not obey his commands. A constant feature is that the harder the musician tries to correct the problem, the worse it becomes. One must counsel against such strenuous efforts as they are seriously counterproductive.

It is possible that Schumann suffered from this condition which led eventually to his having to give up the piano. The classic account in musicians was given by the famous American pianist, Gary Graffman (Graffman 1986), who described it in vivid detail in one of the early editions of the journal *Medical Problems of Performing Artists*. To quote his own words, he had:

an increasing lack of control of my right hand's fourth and fifth fingers. To begin with I had no pain, no numbness nor any symptom I could possibly explain to a doctor. For all normal purposes, opening jars, tying shoelaces, manipulating chopsticks and even at the piano 99.9% of the time my hand operated as always. It was only in certain extended positions, playing a series of octaves, for example, that my trouble surfaced. I was able to play the first octave normally, but striking each subsequent one caused my fourth finger to draw in more and more, dragging the fifth along with it as the hand contracted and of course hitting the wrong notes. This behavior was in no way affected by fatigue, warming up or good or bad days. Either I could play a certain pattern or I could not. Every time it was exactly the same – an octave span of eight notes of the keyboard is about seven inches, a child could deal with it, but I at fifty was no longer capable of doing so.

Brian Hayes (Hayes 1987), a guitarist, gave a graphic description of his problem. He began inexplicably to miss notes with the right plucking hand, particularly the index finger. Any attempts to flex the index or middle finger at the metaphalangeal (MP) joint caused the ring finger to flex first and with more intensity than he wished. He could not flex the index or middle finger and extend the ring finger at the same time. Without flexing the index, however, the ring finger extensors had full strength. The ring finger would not flex without abduction.

'I couldn't hold the ring finger against the middle and flex the MP joint at the same time. Flexing any finger caused uncontrolled abduction in other fingers. The DIP joints of all four fingers seemed excessively tight.'

The condition almost invariably occurs in mid-career, i.e. when the musician has been playing his instrument for 20 years or more. There is often difficulty with arpeggios or broken octaves at the piano or double stops on the violin. Speed may then be lost during percussive passages and where there are rapid alternating ascending or descending patterns of notes. The finger begins to tighten and 'cramps up' and then aching and fatigue is felt in the forearm. In Brandfonbrener's series (Brandfonbrener 1995), the average age of onset was 38. In her series of 58 cases, carefully followed, there were 17 woodwind players, 16 keyboard players, 15 string players, 7 brass players and 3 percussionists.

Twenty-five musicians have been diagnosed as having dystonia in our central clinic in the last 3 years: five pianists, all with inco-ordination of middle ring finger or little fingers, four of whom were referred on for neurological check-up; four guitarists, three with left index finger problems; four bass guitarists; two accordion players with right index or middle finger problems; one each oboist, flautist, cellist, drummer, saxophonist and banjo player and three trombonists, one horn player and one trumpeter with embouchure.

Lederman (Lederman 1987) has written extensively on this condition and tabulated 14 string players whom he studied who had a whole variety of dystonic manifestations. These could be the middle ring or little fingers, the index or middle fingers, middle finger alone, ring finger alone, thumb alone or a combination of some or all of these – but the pattern for each individual patient is almost always the same.

Curiously, there may be a mirror image effect, for when the patient simulates the playing of the instrument with his unaffected hand (Lockwood 1992), dystonic movements and cramp will appear in the resting affected hand, thus indicating that this must be a central lesion. Eventually the dystonic problems can spread to activities of daily life, but in the early stages and indeed for quite a long time the patient finds that ordinary activities are completely unaffected. These patients may even have cramps on the piano but be able to play the violin without any trouble or type without problems. Patients do not complain of pain or tremor or paraesthesiae. The problem is simply one of lack of control of fine movements, painless inco-ordination, disobedience of the digit or inability to blow a note correctly on a wind instrument.

A familial background has been described. One patient, a twin, had typical writers' cramp. The other twin had various combinations of central tremor, primary writing tremor and writers' cramp. Another pair of identical twins have also been described who were separated at a very young age and were educated far apart. Both became professional musicians and both separately developed focal dystonias (Altenmuller 1998).

Brandfonbrener described precipitating or contributory factors to the onset of dystonia in her 58 patients. In 19 there was no discernible factor; in 10 there was a sudden increase in playing or practice time; in 8 a radical change in technique; in 7 a return to graduate study after a long time away from the instrument; in 7 trauma, although not particularly recently; in 5 there was nerve entrapment at some stage; in 4 psychological trauma; and in 2 there had been a change of instrument.

Fletcher, Harding and Marsden (Fletcher et al 1991) discussed the relationship between trauma and idiopathic torsion dystonias. They point out that the generalized multifocal or segmental idiopathic torsion dystonias are caused by an autosomal dominant gene with reduced penetrance in about 85% of cases. Of the 104 patients they studied with this types of disorder, 17 gave a history which suggested that dystonic movements had been precipitated or exacerbated by trauma and 8 of these had relatives affected by the condition. They suggest therefore that there may be a hereditary vulnerability to the onset of dystonia which may be precipitated by trauma. Schott (Schott 1985) described a number of patients in which trauma was an antecedent factor and he suggests that damage to a peripheral nerve results in long-term changes in spinal central synaptic mechanisms, a process in dystonia which he compares to that which is well described and understood in causalgia or phantom limb pain. It is now well known that changes in afferent input into the spinal cord can cause marked reorganization in the central nervous system at many levels. He also described (Schott 1983) eight patients initially referred for orthopaedic opinion who subsequently all turned out to have a dystonic disorder. Three of these patients were musicians: a harpist, a violinist and a cellist. In one, the diagnosis of cervical spondylosis and ulnar neuritis had been made, but in fact the condition was a dystonia with curling of the ring and little fingers into the palm. The violinist, who was diagnosed as having cervical spondylosis with shoulder pain, was in fact having difficulty in controlling the bow because of the index finger curling around and inability to control the thumb. Sudden involuntary movements of the middle and ring finger were noticed. The cellist was diagnosed as having a peripheral nerve entrapment neuropathy because of sudden extension movements of the third and fourth finger of the left hand. Eventually this spread to piano-playing and involuntary tremors developed when putting on his coat. Schott suggested that this may well have been a fragment of a more widespread dystonia. Thus diagnosis can be difficult in the early stages, but the point to emphasize is that this disorder is for quite some time entirely painless. These cases highlight the problems which may result from an inaccurate diagnosis which can lead to inappropriate and disastrous surgery.

It is of course essential to exclude local lesions, such as trigger fingers, ganglions and nodular thickening in the palm.

A disorder of inco-ordination of course raises the question of an intracerebral lesion and all of us working in this field have seen from time to time patients who have presented with dystonia and who have turned out to have a meningioma or other intracerebral space-occupying lesion. It is therefore imperative to make a full neurological examination and to refer for further investigations those patients where there is the slightest suggestion of any other neurological symptom or sign, and it is probably wise so to do in the early stages of dystonia. Most patients present when the condition is well established and the longer it has been present the less likely is there to be a structural cause.

Tubiana and his physiotherapist, Chamagne, have for many years made a carefully detailed study of this condition (Tubiana and Chamagne, 1983, 1993). They have developed a classification, which Tubiana outlines later in this chapter, which is very useful for follow-up purposes and gives some indication of the probable prognosis.

Recent research suggests that focal dystonia is a disorder of reciprocal innervation and Bain (Bain 1998) has shown, by electrical studies, that the second phase of inhibition, the presynaptic phase, is abnormal and mirrors very well the

findings described in writers' cramp. Others believe that it is a disorder of central control at a high level, possibly of the basal ganglia.

Altenmuller (Altenmuller 1998) believes that dystonia in musicians may be related to the specific sensory motor skills uniquely demanded of string and wind players. He had found that in 30% of musician patients dystonia might extend to writers' cramp or one of the more generalized dystonic states such as blepharospasm or spasmodic torticollis. He believes that the lesion is in the Supplementary Association Motor Area (SAMA) and premotor area and is primarily a disorder of *preparation for* a motor skill. It is not felt that this is incompatible with Bain's finding of a disorder of presynaptic inhibition, probably due to a lesion of the basal ganglia. The SAMA lesion may focus itself on the basal ganglia, thus causing the peripheral disorder.

The Feldenkreis technique can be helpful – in this modality the patient learns control by starting with very simple movements and gradually building up to more complex ones once having learnt to relax and control muscle activity (Nelson 1989). Yang Huayu (1996) described two young musicians in whom the dystonia was cured by psychotherapy, but these cases came on at a much earlier age than one normally associates with the condition and there were very clear-cut psychodynamic problems. Usually in the mature adult musician there is little or no evidence of psychological disturbance other than the natural frustration and depression caused by the inability to play. The condition appears to be a kind of fatigue of the control system of complex movement patterns as a result of prolonged use. It is of course essential to establish whether there are any precipitating factors, such as a change of instrument, a change in technique, previous trauma or emotional disturbance.

Butler (Butler 1998) described the North East English Initiative in Management of Dystonia. The incidence of dystonia was found in an epidemiological survey to be 42.25 per 100 000 persons. He had pioneered the initiative of a dystonia nurse practitioner who visited patients in their homes and, when appropriate, gave therapy, including botulinum toxin, reassurance and psychological support. He hoped that some day a musician with a national reputation would 'come out' and admit to the problem. This would allow musicians to confess to their disorder and seek help much earlier.

Botulinum toxin has proved valuable in severe dystonia but the dose needs to be repeated regularly as reinnervation takes place (Cole et al 1991). However, its use in musicians has been abandoned by most serious workers as it inevitably leads to weakness, albeit temporary, and prevents proper performance. It is also too imprecise, since it is very difficult to localize a single musculotendinous unit in the forearm flexor mass.

Certainly the approach should be holistic – one with correction of any obvious locomotor problems, particularly around the shoulder girdle, by instituting a technique of relaxation and body control and careful assessment of playing technique, lifestyle and any relevant psychosocial and emotional factors. Professor Carola Grindea (Grindea 1996) has claimed success with a number of pianists by stressing freedom of wrist movement and correcting proximal muscle tension (see Chapter 3).

All authorities in this field recognize that the earlier the condition is diagnosed, the more likely the patient is to respond to this multidisciplinary approach. Those in whom the condition has persisted for a long time and are in the lowest of the Tubiana grades are never likely to return to professional playing, but may be able to teach.

Incidence: classification of severity and results of therapy

Raoul Tubiana

About 400 cases of upper extremity focal dystonia have been referred to our unit. Most of them were professional instrumentalists.

Dystonia is predominant in men. The average age of onset in our series was 38 years. Similar gender and age distribution have been reported by Hochberg (Hochberg et al 1990) and by Lederman (Lederman 1991). It is interesting to note that this distribution is different in misuse/overuse syndrome in which women outnumber men and the average age is younger (in our series 25 years at the onset for women).

Piano and string players predominate: 142 pianists, 105 guitarists, 86 violinists, 8 violists, 8 cellists and bassists, 4 accordionists, 2 harpists,

10 percussionists, but only a limited number of woodwind and brass players (8 oboists, 7 clarinetists, 5 flautists, 3 saxophonists and 1 bassoonist). This may be because of our specialization in upper limb surgery. We even had to treat three conductors.

In pianists, there is a prevalence of focal dystonia in the right hand (70%). Ulnar digits are more frequently involved on the right side, radial digits on the left side. In guitarists there is also a prevalence on the right side. The long, ring and index fingers are more frequently involved, on the right hand, the index and the ring fingers on the left hand. The thumb is rarely involved on both sides. In violinists, the left side is the most frequently involved: 72% against 28% on the bowing arm. We have seen three cases of focal dystonia with peribuccal muscle contractions in woodwind players (embouchure).

In the majority of our cases of focal dystonia in musicians, the abnormal movements appear only during playing on the occasion of one specific act, often when playing rapid passages. Usually the absence of motor control in the musician is limited to the fingers and sometimes the wrist, but there is no progression of the disorder to other parts of the body. However, in rare cases we have noticed an extension of the disorder to the wrist or dystonic movements in the proximal part of the limb. Also, we have found on rare occasions familial dystonic disorders such as writers' cramp or torticollis.

Pain is rarely present at the beginning but in many patients increases progressively, probably due to painful contractions of muscles. However, in most of our dystonic musicians, these disorders of co-ordination are painless.

In all our dystonic patients, we have found the existence of vicious postures of the upper limb, extending to the shoulder girdle and the spine, and when playing, movements that do not respect normal physiology such as hyperflexion with radial deviation of the wrist or hyperpronation of the hand. Therefore, because of our orthopaedic outlook we decided to correct these defects empirically. Since 1965 Philippe Chamagne (Chamagne 1986) has been in charge of re-education and he has progressively developed a therapeutic programme which consists of making the patient aware of his poor posture, deprogramming non-physiological postures and then teaching new movements that respect normal physiology. Re-education is not restricted to the upper limb and includes the whole body. This treatment is based on relaxation and complete re-education of the neurolomuscular system, for at least a year.

When the musician goes back to use his instrument, return to playing must be very progressive in duration, tempo and complexity and with psychological support. The physiotherapist specializing in the treatment of musicians must have musical knowledge and also psychological sensitivity to understand the problems of these artists. When dealing with these special patients, he will not only ensure maintenance of correct posture, but also be aware of the potential problems associated with each specific instrument. As the physiotherapist has intimate contact with the patient from the beginning of the treatment over the long term, he will have a psychological action which is inseparable from the physical rehabilitation.

This empirical treatment that we have instituted had at first no preconceived theoretical basis. J. Decourt (Decourt 1986), Professor of Neurology at the University of Paris, who had the opportunity to examine a certain number of patients treated by Philippe Chamagne, wrote in 1986:

The numerous repetitions of a complex movement in non-physiological conditions, overworking of muscles and nerves, the relentlessness of the patients to overcome problems of high technical ability, all can lead to vicious postures, disharmony between agonist and antagonist muscles and to disorders of proprioceptive sensibility on which depends the functional co-ordination of movements. The professional activity could be, in other words, responsible for imbalance initially and then deformity . . . I had the opportunity to observe some of the remarkable therapeutic results obtained with a long and careful rehabilitation shown by those patients who were treated in this manner.

Assessment of results

At the beginning and at the end of the treatment we use an assessment on a 6-point scale.

0   Unable to play.

1   Plays several notes but stops because of blockage or lack of facility.
2   Plays short sequences without rapidity and with unsteady fingering.
3   Plays easy pieces with restrictions. Rapid sequences stir up motor problems.
4   Nearly normal playing but avoids technically difficult passages for fear of motor problems.
5   Normal playing. Returns to concert performances.

The results at the end of the treatment, evaluated in a group of pianists, violinists and guitarists, has shown the importance of the severity of the dystonia to the success of therapy. Six pianists, four guitarists and one violinist were assessed with grade 0 at the beginning of the treatment: for 11 patients with grade 0, 6 remained at 0. Four pianists had only limited improvement: one moved up to 1, one to 3 and two to 4. One violinist remained at 0. One guitarist with grade 0 moved up to 1.

Of three pianists with grade 1 at the beginning, one moved up to 3 and two to 4. For four guitarists with grade 1, one remained at 1, one moved up to 4 and two to 5. There was no violinist with grade 1.

Of nine pianists with grade 2 at the beginning, three remained at 2, one moved up to 3, two to 4 and two to 5. Of eight violinists with grade 2, three remained at 2, two moved up to 3, one to 4 and two to 5. Of four guitarists with grade 2, one remained at 2 and three moved up to 5.

Of 18 pianists with grade 3, two remained at 2, ten moved up to 4 and six to 5. Of ten violinists with grade 3, one remained at 3, two moved up to 4 and seven to 5. Of eight guitarists with grade 3, three moved up to 4 and five to 5.

Of nine pianists with grade 4, one remained at 4 and eight moved up to 5. All the three violinists and the guitarists with grade 4 moved up to 5.

One may conclude that the higher the grade at the beginning, the better the results. Other factors may influence the results such as: the morphological and psychological condition of the musician: in particular, the active participation of the patient in their rehabilitation is essential. This demands an enormous physical and mental effort. The patient's complete collaboration will help towards a successful result. The delay between the onset of the problems and the beginning of the treatment is probably not as important as first thought, as we have seen some patients with dystonic symptoms over several years making a complete recovery. However, a short delay is preferable. Periodic control of posture and movements is mandatory in order to avoid recurrences.

In conclusion, treatment of instrumentalists' focal dystonia is always long and difficult. The results of the treatment depend on the severity of the dystonia, on the quality of the treatment and the collaboration of the patient. The long, comprehensive re-education programme includes the whole body and necessitates the unswerving and dedicated participation of the patient. It is a teamwork based on confidence. Most of our patients had already undergone several types of treatment with no obvious benefit. Cole (Cole et al 1991) stated 'focal dystonia in a musician is characterized both by spasms and a disorder of co-ordination. Improvement in the spasms can be accomplished with botulinium toxin injection, but the motor co-ordination is not addressed with the treatment'. Focal dystonia formerly thought to be of psychogenic origin in reality is due to disturbances in fine motor control. Encouraging results obtained by our method of correction of postural defects associated with re-education of movements that respect normal physiology seems to emphasize the role of peripheral factors in the onset of focal dystonia in musicians. However, we don't yet know the pathogenesis of this condition.

In our opinion, relaxation techniques or local injections may, in certain cases, be used as an adjuvant, but the basis of therapy is a re-education programme.

References

Altenmuller E (1998) Causes and cures of focal limb dystonia in musicians. Proceedings of the International Congress of Musicians: Health and the Musician, York 1997. British Association of Performing Art Medicine: London.

Bain P (1998) Reciprocal inhibition of the median nerve H-reflex in musicians with painless incoordination syndromes: evidence for an occupational dystonia. Proceedings of the International Congress of Musicians: Health and the Musician, York 1998. British Association of Performing Art Medicine: London.

Brandfonbrener AG (1995) Musicians with focal dystonia. *Med Probl Perform Artists* **10**:121–27.

Butler AG (1998) The working life of musicians: a survey into dystonia in North East England. Proceedings of the International Congress of Musicians: Health and the Musician, York 1998. British Association of Performing Art Medicine: London.

Chamagne Ph (1986) Les 'crampes fonctionelles' ou 'dystonies de fonction' chez les écrivains et les musiciens. *Ann Chir Main* **5**(2):148–52.

Cole RA, Cohen LG, Hallet M (1991) Treatment of musician's cramp with botulinium toxin. *Med Probl Perform Artists* **6**:137–43.

Decourt J (1986) Commentaires sur l'article de Ph. Chamagne: Les 'crampes fonctionelles' ou 'dystonies de fonction' chez les écrivains et les musiciens. *Ann Chir Main* **5**(2):152.

Fletcher NA, Harding AE, Marsden CD (1991) The relationship between trauma and idiopathic torsion dystonia. *Journal of Neurol Neurosurg Psychiatry* **54**:713–17.

Graffman G (1986) Doctor can you lend an ear? *Med Probl Perform Artists* **1**:3.

Hayes B (1987) Painless hand problems of string pluckers. *Med Probl Perform Artists* **2**:39–40.

Hochberg F, Harris SU, Blattert TR (1990) Occupational hand cramps: professional disorders of motor control. *Hand Clin* **6**:417–28.

Huaya Y (1996) Psychothérapie et dyskinésie chez les musiciens. *Medicine des Arts* **16**:13–15.

Lederman RJ (1987) Occupational cramp in instrumental musicians. *Med Probl Perform Artists* **3**:45–50.

Lederman RJ (1991) Focal dystonia in instrumentalists: clinical features. *Med Probl Perform Artists* **6**:132–6.

Lockwood AM (1992) Focal dystonic movements provoked by use of the unaffected hand. *Mirror Movement Dystonia* **7**:22–4.

Nelson SH (1989) Playing with the entire self: the Feldenkreis method and musicians. *Seminar Neurol* **9**:97.

Schott GD (1983) The idiopathic dystonias. A note on their orthopaedic presentation. *J Bone Joint Surg* **65B**:51–7.

Schott GD (1985) The relationship of peripheral trauma and pain to dystonia. *J Neurol* **48**:698.

Schott GD (1986) Induction of involuntary movements by peripheral trauma: an analogy with causalgia. *Lancet* **27**:712.

Tubiana R, Chamagne Ph (1983) Crampes profes-sionelles du membre supérieur. *Ann Chir Main* **2**:134–42.

Tubiana R, Chamagne Ph (1993) Les affections profes-sionelles du membre supérieur chez les musiciens. *Bull Acad Med* **177**:203–16.

15
The musical temperament

Christopher B Wynn Parry

While sports psychology and the psychology of the sportsman has received much attention and wide publicity, the psychology of the musician has had virtually no public attention. After all we are considering a person who has mastered an incredibly complex art over decades, requiring extraordinary manual or vocal dexterity and an ability to blend with other players, listen to his or her own playing as well as that of those around and cover enormous ranges of style and techniques. Moreover, they have to put themselves before the public night after night with little rest or cosseting from trainers, coaches or psychologists and, unlike the sportsman, who is allowed failure, must always get it right. Fortunately, very recently a start has been made. A number of musical psychologists have made in-depth studies of the characteristics and make-up of musicians' personalities and how they differ amongst each other relative to their instruments (Kemp 1996).

What sort of person then is the musician? And how can a profounder understanding of their characteristics help caring professions provide support when they are ill? Various researches indicate that most musicians are introverted, so there is a tendency to direct energy inwards, resulting in a reserved temperament. They are shown to have considerable resourcefulness, self-sufficiency and personal inner strengths. They are able to tolerate long periods of solitude for practice. This is perceived as boring and monotonous by the extroverted, but they can suffer from overstimulation and their performances can deteriorate more rapidly under higher stress conditions. They share with other creative types a degree of independence and ability to be analytical about their work. They have a high level of sensitivity, imagination and intuition. As Myers (Myers 1993) puts it, they have feelings that are deep but seldom

expressed because the inner tenderness and passionate conviction are both masked by reserve and repose. These feelings are on the whole not projected outwards, but are kept private, thus concealing the very thing that motivates them most highly. This may be responsible in part for their high levels of anxiety.

Their background is unique, involving having taken up this difficult art at an early age, being perceived as special by their parents, spending long hours in solitary practice. They have been to special schools with the well-known hothouse effect, have been denied a normal social and sporting milieu and have had to work hard throughout their school and college career.

As Kemp explains, their high level of anxiety is connected with their investment of so much of themselves in what may be a precarious future. The deep feelings of being different, their continual striving for perfection, vulnerability in a performing situation, the uncertainties and competitiveness of their lives, the irregular hours and disturbed social life all make for potential anxiety. It is not uncommon for children who take up an instrument seriously, to be bullied, particularly when that instrument is not seen as appropriate for their sex by the crowd, e.g. violin or flute for boys or trombone for girls, and this can have a long-lasting effect on their psyche.

Several workers have identified stereotyped patterns of interpersonal perceptions. String players saw brass players as heavy drinkers, lacking refinement, with lower intelligence and noisy behaviour, and interestingly brass players themselves claim to be gregarious, loud, confident and jovial. The brass saw the string players as frustrated, quiet and feminine. The string players saw themselves as sensitive, competitive, neurotic and insecure. String playing is particularly complex, with the interrelation of finger, wrist and arm movements and overall posture, with very acute aural skills and sensitivity to pitch and nuance. There is a profound sense of communication between the player and the instrument. Jacqueline du Pré described the cello as her friend and could not bear to be parted from it when on holiday as a child. String players tend not to mix widely, forming close relationships with one or two people only. Cellists were found to be particularly introverted. Brass players, of course, have a marked degree of exposure. They have nowhere to hide when an error has been made. They have not the mass of colleagues to hide among like string players, and as the music has to go on they have to have a high degree of self-confidence. Unlike other musicians, brass players do not have visual cues for playing the musical notes. They have to depend entirely on their lips and ears and have to imagine the notes aurally. They are found to be more extrovert and less sensitive than string players.

Yet, mirabile dictu, the musician is a versatile and resilient person. In Danziger's (1997) survey of 51 musicians in the London Symphony Orchestra, 30 were still in love with their profession and were totally dedicated to it. Of these, 6 had marital problems, 7 suffered chronic fatigue, 8 were fed-up with their lifestyle and 5 had regular stage fright, but of all of these only 3 wanted to give it all up and all said they would do the same again.

Pop musicians suffer many stresses and have above-average levels of anxiety. In a recent survey it was reported that 54% found humour the most valued corrective. Taking exercise and talking problems through with a friend came high on the list. There was no evidence that rock/pop musicians smoke or drank excessively more frequently than the normal population (Wills and Cooper 1988).

Havas (Havas 1986) asked the interesting question why it is that Hungarian gypsy players appear to be immune to stage fright and performance anxiety. She believes that first of all they are not burdened with the responsibilities of a social system. They do not have to do better than their fellows in order to succeed. In fact, she said, they would be hard-pressed to understand why anyone wanted to succeed at all. Their sole interest is in the pleasure of the listeners. They are free from all obligations except one – to communicate their passion for the music.

Stage fright and anxiety

The artist performer is a unique and sensitive person requiring continuous physical and mental effort to maintain the standard of excellence which musicians constantly demand of themselves. Psychological profiles carried out on musicians show that they are particularly affected by insecurities and have a combination of self-criticism and insecurity which leads to anxiety.

It is well recognized that musicians tend to somatize more than any other group of the population (Miller and Kupersmuti 1990). This is hardly surprising considering that their whole art and performance depends on the use of their body, and should something go wrong with either their mood or their physical state, somatic symptoms are highly likely to result and can present with muscular aches and pains.

Where it is universally accepted that a certain degree of nervous tension is good, indeed essential, for a high-quality performance, an excessively nervous state can lead to severe problems. Stage fright is defined as the artist's fear of audiences and auditions and it may even happen in rehearsals if this involves particular musical exposure. Andy Evans, the leading arts psychologist in this field (see Chapter 16), has written a brilliant book on musical confidence which points out that causes can be many and varied.

The French psychologist Fresnel has pointed out that there are many 'tracs' (fears), not one. In her study 99% of 72 singers and comedians confessed to stage fright (Fresnel and Bourgault 1996). According to Schultz 58% of the Vienna Symphony Orchestra had stage fright, (Schultz 1981) and 72% of London orchestral players had anxiety at some stage which affected their performance, as reported by Ian James in Chapter 17; in 25% it was chronic and troublesome. There seems to be, however, a lesser incidence on the Continent which may reflect the better conditions of artistic careers. Fresnel's study found that in 12% of cases there was a depressive component in addition to stage fright, particularly among singers. In 22% there was an additional phobia, fear of flying, claustrophobia, fear of spiders, snakes or mice. The 'trac' usually began early on in the career, before the first audition, competition or first public performance. Andy Evans (see Chapter 16) points out that stage fright is a learned response and that there is often a trigger factor that initiated the problem and must be carefully sought. It may have started in childhood: parental fear or anxiety can be transferred to a child. Often there has been a dramatic background. He quotes a violinist who was required to play in a string quartet performing in a school play at the top of a tower. She was terrified of heights and it was moreover a cold day. She froze up and ruined her part. From that time on she had a feeling of panic whenever she had to perform in public. It was the drama, not the music, that was relevant in this example. Sara Bernhart remarked to a young comedian who boasted of not feeling stage fright, 'Don't worry it will come as your talent develops'. Quite apart from the fear of presenting oneself as an artist and performer to a public, the music profession itself is well known to be viciously competitive and highly insecure. Berlioz remarked that 'La musique est divine mais l'orchestre est merde'.

It is customary to categorize the clinical picture of stage fright into three aspects: first, physical symptoms with increased heart rate, sweating, increased rate of breathing, dry mouth, lack of appetite, nausea and stomach upsets including diarrhoea and vomiting. Second, cognitive reactions, feelings of loss of control, loss of musical memory, sense of catastrophic anticipation of failing. Third, behavioural disorders, cancelling performances, drinking too much, faking playing, walking off stage.

Andy Evans in his management of stage fright introduces positive coping strategies:

I feel nervous, my desk partner is putting me off my playing. He has always been critical of me. My bow arm is unsteady. I am sure I will start to shake and my bow will jump.

will be replaced by:

I could play this perfectly well when I practised this morning. I am here because I am good. I am thought by others to be a good player. In fact when I think about it, I am better than he is. He has got a problem, I haven't. I shall play fine.

Obviously mastery of the technical side of the performance and the emotional qualities of the music is essential, and during practice the opportunity is taken to rehearse positive imaging.

Part of the strategy lies in divorcing panic from the situation in which it originally arose so that the player appreciates that it is not a musical cause per se. In general one aims to reduce fear to manageable proportions, narrowing down anxiety to one specific. One must remind oneself that one has coped well in the past. The adage 'You are only as good as your last performance' is rubbish. One should adopt the view that it's business as usual. A few wrong notes is compatible with an adequate performance – and will anyone actually notice? Challenge is an essential part of life and it is to be welcomed. One can turn the physical symptoms into a positive feature: increased heart rate shows that I am well hyped up and does not at all spell disaster.

Performance anxiety is much commoner than generally appreciated. It is always wise to ask if it is causing problems as help can readily be given.

Beta blockers

These drugs are certainly helpful for they diminish or abolish the physiological body responses already discussed, thus they will slow the heart rate, reduce sweating and diminish tremor. In Fresnel's group, 45% found relaxation helpful, 16% smoked or drank, while 27% had no strategies, 5% used beta blockers and only 1% used anxiolytics – most found they would reduce dexterity and fine control and quickly abandoned them. These are in any case to be regarded as a rescue operation for emergencies, for it is generally accepted now that whenever possible cognitive behavioural therapy as described is far better than drugs. Although the drugs reduce the physiological effects of stress, they do not get at the cause. Now that counselling is becoming more freely available and arts psychologists are becoming intimately involved in musicians' problems, this approach is always preferred. There are certain dangers inherent in these drugs, in particular they should never be given if the patient has a history of asthma, and it is always wise for them to be prescribed by an experienced physician who understands musicians.

Catherine Butler (Butler 1996), an arts psychologist, has carried out some important research into the problems posed by music students and the sorts of stress that they experience. She has delineated the profile of those that are likely to break down. She found that those who had the mysterious quality of ego strength survived best, with high self-esteem, musical obsession and independence. Those who succumbed to stress, presenting with depression and very often musculoskeletal symptoms, were found to have low self-esteem and confidence, they saw their siblings as rivals and worried about critical or anxious mothers and somewhat distant fathers. They project these unsatisfactory relationships on to the conservatoire and the people in it. They are reluctant to seek help, nervous of committing themselves totally to their career, suffer poor health, have few friends and see their peers as competitors and not colleagues. They feel isolated, are uncomfortable practising and have a very high incidence of performance anxiety.

In contrast, she points out that successful students get on well with their siblings, have a happy parental background, both parents playing or singing and having a very relaxed and affectionate adult relationship. The students have confidence to ask to change their professor if necessary and enjoy the excitement of performance. They aspire to be professionals, and if they cannot do so they are prepared to choose another form of art or join the caring professions.

Butler makes a plea for the conservatoires to help the student complete the process of adolescent emotional separation from the mother and she feels the organization of conservatoires needs to be reviewed so there is better communication with the pupils. It is important, she says, that the year the young musician spends at the conservatoire, which is in effect a very small proportion in a very long process of artistic growth, should allow for the artist's consciousness to regulate their development at its natural pace. She believes that much can be done to prevent these problems, and that it should be possible to prevent stressed students becoming ill and dropping out by testing all new students to discover those potentially at risk, those who are at risk being given the opportunity of counselling to acquire a self-awareness which would prevent their suffering.

Nigel Kennedy, in a television programme on musical prodigies, pointed to the monstrous lifestyle in which the young prodigy is involved and refers to this as a circus ring. What happens in the prodigy's future when he or she burns out and what happens to those who are brought up to be prodigies and then fail? The tragic story of a brilliant pianist, Terence Judd, who committed suicide should be a warning to all.

The Juillard School has recently introduced a comprehensive counselling service, well described by Kanefield in 1990. They found that 12.5% of music students avail themselves of the psychological services. Common problems the students faced were concern about their identity, self-esteem, self-expression and body image. Others included problems of relationships, separation from and loss of family members and general instability in relationships with most people, the effects of traumatic events such as death and abuse, worry about themselves, their career and future, performing anxiety and depression.

There is no doubt that psychological and emotional problems are a very real cause of stress in music students and that an understanding of this situation and prompt treatment is all important to prevent chronic morbidity in later life.

References

Butler C (1996) Stress and the music student. *ISM Music Journal* **1**:246–8.

Danziger D (1997) *The Orchestra. Lives Behind the Music.* HarperCollins: London.

Fresnel EE, Eltaz E, Bourgault R (1996) Voix et trac stress anxiete de performance. *Medecin des Arts* **18**:3–6.

Havas K (1986) Stage fright – its causes and cures with special reference to violin playing. Bosworth: London.

Kanefield EL (1990) Psychological services at the Juillard School. *Med Probl Perform Artists* **5**:41–4.

Kemp AE (1996) *The Musical Temperament: Psychology and Personality of Musicians.* Oxford University Press: Oxford.

Muller DK, Kupersmuti JR (1990) Louisville-Pach psychiatric problems of performing artists. *Med Probl Perform Artists* **5**:19–22.

Myers IB (1993) Gifts differing: *Understanding Personality Type*. Consulting Psychologists Press: Palo Alto, California.

Shultz W (1981) Analysis of a symphony orchestra. Sociological and sociopsychological aspects. In:

Pipatee M, ed. *Stress and Music*. Wilhelm Braumuller: Vienna.

Wills G, Cooper CL (1988) *Pressure Sensitive*. Sage Publications: London.

16
Performance psychology and the musician's hand

Andy Evans

The importance of the hand in human psychology is reflected in many expressions, such as 'get a grip', 'pull all the stops out', 'pull one's finger out', 'lay hands on', 'treat with a firm hand', and 'have one's hands tied'. 'Fingering' is vital to instrumental technique, 'grip' is a key feature of bowing, hand or baton movements are the essence of conducting – only singers are exempt from the need to employ the hand in music-making. The focus on the hand in music-making is consequently so absolute that any technical or physical malfunction hits at the heart of the musician's self-confidence, and is easily exaggerated and dramatized into a more global 'problem' which may occupy the forefront of the musician's mind until both physical and psychological difficulties are resolved.

Residual worries may include 'curses' acquired from parents or teachers, feelings of hands being 'naughty' or 'disobedient' (still the word used for dystonias), sometimes reinforced in childhood by a sharp crack of the ruler from our more sadistic piano teachers. There are further all the feelings of technical inadequacy associated with self-learned fingerings on guitar and piano, and the constant search for speed, for which the lightning-fingered Eric Clapton was ironically nicknamed 'Slow Hand', from 'slow hand clap'(ton). Hand speed is to the instrumentalist what high notes are to the singer – a potentially alarming signal that the maximum possible feats of technique have to be accomplished, and fear of inadequate speed and dexterity are never totally out of mind.

A further psychological dimension is how the musician 'maps' his musical imagination. Some musicians rely on sound from their first contact with an instrument, and map their musical world – as jazz musicians do – by shifts in chord and melody, so the fingers obey the sound. Classical musicians routinely rely on the printed score for their mapping – the fingers obey the score. Other musicians, like guitarists and drummers, map their musical thought in terms of finger movements, hand positions and hand movements, and their tablatures reflect this.

While musical technique is aural (for sounds), visual (for cues) and kinetic (for movements), it originates in the musical brain, which varies greatly from one musician to another. While one pianist preparing for a major competition may use a high-planning, low-risk/low-gain strategy of rehearsing precise movements, another may go for a higher excitement level by spontaneously imaging the flow of the musical argument in each performance and hoping that the all-round technique will allow the hand to follow where the brain leads, to the ultimate goal of the elusive 'peak performance experience' musicians so cherish. Such was Alfred Cortot, who would rehearse 20 ways of playing a passage and then play the twenty-first when he went on stage.

So the way the hand is 'programmed' by the brain is of vital importance to the final quality of performance. Accepted wisdom is that the imagination rules the hand, not vice versa. In terms of practice, this ideally means that the musician practises 'musical thinking' as conveyed through tone and technique. Overuse–misuse problems may indicate that fingerwork is being pursued in an obsessive or ritualistic way which affords little 'musical' pleasure or progress, leading to loss of motivation or actual physical problems. A cautionary tale is that of Schumann, who ritually pursued finger independence to the point of having to abandon being a virtuoso – though this personal blunder thankfully enriched the world of musical composition.

Frequently encountered problems of instrumentalists

String players

The violin is a masterpiece of bad engineering. Not only is it difficult to hold under the chin, but the right-hand bowing action is a perfect example of awful human ergonomics. Given the starting premise that performers are prone to hand shake due to the effects of adrenalin flow induced by confronting a large audience and a further ordeal by fire from their peers, section leaders and conductors, the very last thing they want to hold in a shaking hand is a metre-long wooden object which will go through a motion of several centimetres at the opposite end of a minute hand movement of a few millimetres. It is hardly surprising that string players refer to stage fright as 'the shakes'. In consequence, the performance psychologist makes friends with large quantities of our national violin sections. The same is true of violists to a lesser extent, and so down the descending scale to cellists and bassists, who suffer considerably less as the bow gets shorter, heavier and lower in grip, and so present in increasingly infrequent numbers. Less often, violinists present with left-hand problems involving vibrato. If wrongly applied this can lead to overuse–misuse syndrome, which is dealt with below.

Wind and brass

Wind players are more rarely seen for hand shake – there is no bow and the hand is conveniently on the keys. Even the embouchure is less shake prone, particularly in the case of the clarinet. Brass players are beset with embouchure problems – particularly the horns – but hand problems are again a relative rarity.

Keyboards

The primary problem of concert pianists is the fear of memory lapses. Having said that, performance nerves do affect hand technique through shaking and sweating, and if this is the case treatment for a general reduction in anxiety should be undertaken by the psychologist. Where the problem is overuse–misuse syndrome, this is dealt with below.

Plucked instruments

Both guitarists and banjo players are prone to dystonia and overuse–misuse syndrome. This tends to be in the 'plucking hand' i.e. the right hand if right-handed, and may occur in cases where either a plectrum is used or the fingers pluck the strings.

Percussion

Percussionists may suffer overuse–misuse syndrome as their fellow musicians do, and have added technical worries like overhand/underhand choices of grip and the whole question of how and where to practise, and how to avoid boredom when using practice pads rather than the real kit for reasons of noise.

Problems of psychological loss of function

The early literature of Freud contains some classic accounts of 'hysterical conversions', notably that of Anna O., where there was a somatization including some loss of hand function following the traumatic death of her father (Freud and Breuer 1974). Freud's conclusion that where there is inadequate emotional reaction and working through of a trauma such as death, the outlet for expression might be through the body, is equally true to this day.

I had such a case of a guitarist who, following the death of his father, which had not been worked through, had a sudden loss of right-hand dexterity on stage in the presence of a 'father figure' whom he had looked up to musically. This loss of dexterity was not present in practice, but continued to occur on stage, and through working through the events of the time he was able to fully recover his hand function.

Treating problems of psychological loss of function

Cases less 'classic' than the above can also be usefully treated by the same methods, though in some more paradoxical cases of arm and hand problems the origin remains stubbornly rooted in the unconscious. The patient may not see the utility of pursuing a longer process of sleuthing round the unconscious when the apparent problem is physical, and a frequently heard plea is 'Can't you send me to a hypnotist who will root it out and cure me in a few sessions?'. The image is closer to that of the vaudeville stage hypnotist than the clinical hypnotherapist, whose attempts to teach self-hypnosis and professionally examine the root causes appear to cause a severe let-down of expectations.

Provided that a good working relationship is established to achieve some psychological benefits, progress does take place, and after a while patients I have seen have recovered most or all of their hand function. The timescale, however, may be over a year – not the quick fix they had in mind at first.

One alternative for the brave psychologist is simply to bluff it out and refuse to collude with the problem. Provided the psychologist acts with extreme authority and directiveness this may work, as it did when Freud treated the conductor Bruno Walter for a difficulty in conducting with the baton. He carefully directed Walter to take a holiday in Sicily for a definite period of time, stating with absolute certainty that the problem would disappear on his return, which it did. While few mere mortals would be so authoritative, the lesson in not colluding with the problem is the foundation of modern pain management and is well learned.

Problems of physical loss of function

Dystonia

Because the dystonias typically involve no pain or total loss of function, they are less dramatic in presentation than overuse–misuse syndrome. Nonetheless, they are a real problem in that any fault in technique affects a perfect performance, and consequently the livelihood of the sufferer. The performance psychologist may help with alternative techniques designed to bypass or 'fool' the problem, because the paradoxical nature of dystonias may lend itself to strategic solutions. General reduction in psychological tension and life stressors may help either directly or indirectly, and a programme of ignoring rather than obsessively colluding with the dystonia may again help. This is not an easy area to operate in, and advances in research will help considerably with our limited understanding of how to diagnose and treat this problem.

Overuse–misuse syndrome (RSI)

What is often referred to as 'RSI' seems on the face of it to fit the cases of workers such as keyboard operators, and has thus been seen by the various unions protecting the working conditions of journalists and other frequent keyboard operators as being simply 'overuse'. This interpretation was originally used for pianists, violinists and guitarists in which it is most often seen. Performing arts specialists dispute this and claim it is better interpreted as not only 'overuse' but also 'misuse' of the body – particularly resulting from practising for long periods in a psychological and physical state of stress and inappropriate posture, for instance before important exams, auditions and competitions.

The difference in emphasis is important not only for diagnosis but also for prevention and treatment. The treatment for 'overuse' is considered to be complete rest, while that for 'misuse' is much more complex, including psychological help with stress reduction, practice attitudes and posture correction.

Whatever the interpretation, the initial treatment plan requires prompt intervention by a medical specialist, in conjunction with a physical/postural specialist (usually a physiotherapist), which should serve to diagnose the nature and extent of the problem and the overall nature of the treatment plan; it may go on to involve the psychologist and possibly also any of the following, as needed and appropriate:

• An Alexander or Feldenkreis technique practitioner

- An osteopath
- An acupuncturist
- A hypnotherapist.

A coherent treatment plan is essential not only for the correct treatment of the problem, but crucially to gain the patient's confidence in the recovery plan that is to be put in place. Without one 'centralized' team approach, the patient will show every desire to 'browse' around all sorts of plausible practitioners, each of whom will point out both the 'perceived' focus of the problem and a 'helpful' intervention. If no attempt is made to co-ordinate the treatments offered, the patient will rapidly end up substantially out of pocket, totally confused and mistrustful of everyone involved in the 'alleged' solution of the problem.

Since the psychologist will rarely be the first practitioner involved in a case of physical pain, it is crucial that those involved in the initial assessment present a realistic picture of what the psychologist can and cannot do, so that the patient comes to therapy sessions with the right attitude. An example of the 'wrong' attitude results from a referral to a psychologist which goes along the lines of 'I'll send you to Mr X, who is very good with musicians and will surely help sort out the problem'. The patient is quite likely to infer that Mr X is, like the medical model just experienced, a person who will give a clear and helpful diagnosis followed by an equally clear recovery plan.

The reality of the psychologist's work is that even assessment is complex – the mind is by far our most complex organ and is not easily examined. Time is required to assemble the jumble of psychological factors potentially involved, and even more time is required to see those factors that stand out as priorities. Yet more time is required for the patient to comprehend and accept his own problem – for the blindingly obvious reason that any material in the 'unconscious' is by definition not yet in the 'conscious' mind. More time again is required for the patient to accept and accommodate changes in perception, attitude and actual behaviour that might eventually help solve a problem or avoid its recurrence. A cherished medical colleague of mine once wryly observed that 'the difference between doctors and psychologists is that with psychologists nobody dies and nobody gets better'. Humour aside, this could well be borne

in mind as an initial approach to the 'softly softly catchy monkey' nature of the psychologist's approach.

In the past I have seen a number of patients who present with less than helpful or realistic attitudes to the work of the psychologist. These are primarily the ideas that:

- Pain is felt 'in the body' so the problem should be in the body
- Physical practitioners therefore seem to offer more of 'a cure'
- 'Talking about' pain is not on the face of it relevant or productive.

Given the high levels of desperation and frustration that musicians feel when contemplating the loss of their life's work and ambitions, this is not surprising, but nor is it helpful. What is helpful is the attitude that mind and body are closely related in a constant feedback loop, and that any gain anywhere in that loop has knock-on gains on the total performance system. Such a holistic attitude may be anathema for the impatient sufferer seeking a clear solution, but it is particularly appropriate in these cases.

Having moved on from some initial 'cautionary advice' on referrals, which has already become second nature to the new corpus of enlightened medical specialists involved in regularly dealing with musicians' problems, we can now look at some of the useful work the psychologist can do with the full co-operation of the correctly referred patient.

Treating overuse–misuse syndrome

The first difficulty both the client and the therapist has to grapple with is 'how much of the pain is physical and how much psychological in origin'. Typically the medical specialist will find some initial problem, e.g. inflammation, and there will be an accompanying diagnosis from a physical practitioner such as 'misalignment', 'bad posture'. No indication is usually given of what percentage of the problem is manufactured in the mind, and indeed such a calculation would be very difficult to achieve. Typically the inflammation improves to the point where nothing shows up on scans, and the postural issues have been dealt with in a number of sessions, with advice for how to use the body better in future. At this point the pain should go away, but in a significant number of cases it does not.

Since the psychologist's initial problem is not knowing exactly what percentage of the problem is physical, the opening premise is that there is no guarantee that he will achieve actual pain reduction. It cannot be too strongly stated that the first task of the psychologist is to get the client's trust that talking will be of some use. This trust may be given and then withdrawn according to whether 'results' occur, i.e. the perception of pain lessens. The psychologist is therefore well advised to start with an overview of how talking might prove useful. He may outline some of the following possible areas of help.

- Desensitizing the mind to pain. One enlightened GP described (to a patient of mine) the main function of the brain as 'ignoring things'. This useful advice – that the brain would cease to function if it were not able to prioritize what needed to be attended to – goes a long way towards describing the necessity of persuading the brain to ignore pain rather than 'noticing it' constantly. Even where organic function is restored, the image of pain can linger, because it obeys the laws of classical conditioning laid down by Pavlov – rapid onset, followed by slow desensitization. Pain is no longer actual but a dramatically over-sensitized perception, which the brain is unable to let go of. The psychologist's role here is in facilitating this process of desensitization.
- Loss of function, and the emotional stages of loss.
- Careers advice if and where the medical advice is complete rest.
- Tendency to hypochondria, which musicians are particularly prone to because of their heightened imagination, sense of drama, self-involvement and non-verbal focus.
- Dealing with sabotage. Performers 'pushed' into a career on stage, e.g. by parents, may physically break down as a defensible way of opting out and preserving their identities and alternative career goals.
- Dealing with perfectionism. This is a personality type that seems prone to physical breakdown. Since high stress is invested in being perfect, there may be a tendency to overpractise or practise obsessively and unproductively. The standards for such perfection may be set by parents, or siblings and peers for whom there is a high degree of envy and obsessive competition, or by artistic role models (Heifetz and the equivalent) one strives to emulate. The most imaginative artists can even create a nearly-believed-in perfect fantasy version of themselves, incorporating envied physical and mental features of others, which becomes more and more dissociated from their real values and attributes. I have found by examining my database of personality profiles that the most successful performers I have seen are normal or even low on perfectionism, while those who have dropped out or had psychosomatic problems score extremely high. There is a crucial difference between performing a task perfectly, which is the kind of technical mastery successful performers have, and trying to live up to an 'image' of being perfect, which is where the problems start.

Personal injury

Personal injury is something I dealt with regularly for 2 years as an occupational psychologist in rehabilitation centres, and then later on occasions in my ordinary practice. The overwhelming lesson I learned was that of totally separating the roles of the forensic psychologist, whose job is to fight the corner of the injured party in court as an expert witness, and that of the confidential counsellor who must on no account get involved in the legal proceedings.

I developed a great deal of sympathy for the inner 'double life' of the victim who is forced over a period of several years simultaneously to maintain a state of injury deserving of compensation and at the same time attempt to recover enough function to carry on with a career as well as possible. This unenviable double life takes an enormous toll on the inner mental state of someone who is grappling with all sorts of stages of loss, with their attendant angers, depressions and utter frustrations.

The services of the best possible forensic psychologist – preferably one who does personal injury cases day in and day out and knows all the legal angles and the most effective lawyers to use – frees the personal counsellor to explore the real personal issues without having to get politically involved and wear two antagonistic hats.

General problems of performance anxiety

Besides the particular psychological factors directly affecting the hand, as outlined above, there is the fact that anything that puts the mind/body continuum of the musician into a state of anxiety is likely adversely to affect various parts of that continuum, resulting for example in shaking of the hand, potential for errors and body and limb stress. Added to this, the psychologist is frequently called in where a hand problem is accompanied by general anxiety about performing, since the incidence of performance anxiety is shown by surveys to be as high as 60–70% in orchestral and freelance musicians.

A full account of techniques for conquering this are outlined in detail in Evans (1994). A brief overview is given below. In my view, the origins of generalized performing anxiety in the musician break down into particular problems, each with different treatments.

Performing anxiety

The classic 'stage fright' is often the result of a sequence of bad experiences. These are frequently 'first time' experiences, such as the first day in school, the first time you had to stand up and recite something to the class from memory, or your first time in the local youth orchestra. Such experiences can 'condition' our behaviour to associate fear and the prospect of failure with performing in public. This is known as a 'learned response'. Such conditioning can either be general, as in feeling a generalized anxiety, or can be a repetitive fear of a particular problem, such as dropping the bow, dropping one's instrument, not being able to pick quickly enough on the guitar, or playing wrong notes.

Treatment consists initially of a cognitive re-evaluation of the musician's beliefs regarding performance, starting with an explanation of the peak in adrenalin response that occurs in all performers (not just those who get anxious) just before until just after going on stage. Persuading the musician that this peak is entirely normal allows him to accept an initial sweating, palpitation and dry mouth as no more than a temporary annoyance that regularly settles down once performance starts. It also soon becomes clear to the musician that he has played through such nerves time and time again, so that the melodramatic feeling of 'panic leading to humiliating failure' can be replaced by a more rational analysis of 'temporary nerves that may slightly compromise but don't prevent performance'.

Treatment then goes on to 'deconstruct' the original fright. Essential steps one must take are to:

- Identify how the panic response became associated with performing in the first place. Take a detailed history including other non-performing panic situations if relevant.
- Begin to dissociate the 'conditioned' panic from the essential process of making music. Monitor performances to identify and deal with the particular 'triggers' the musician is sensitive to.
- Acquire a conscious strategy of mental reactions to respond immediately to recurring triggers.
- Acquire a sense of history and reality: the original 'catastrophe(s)' that caused the panic happened through a freak combination of factors that will not be exactly repeated in normal music-making.
- Acquire a sense of scale: nerves – however unpleasant – are not the same as utter panic. You can play through them and survive them.

Social anxiety

A distinct type of stage fright comes from bad feelings about fellow performers. It is not unknown for orchestral musicians to have nightmares about desk partners or section leaders or to walk off stage in disgust. Some performers are always criticizing others; some feel constantly criticized. Many do both – they feel critical about their own ability and then 'project' this on to others by criticizing them instead. They then feel really bad when they suspect others criticize them. The criticism goes round and round – we dish it out, we take it in.

The world of performance – and classical music in particular – is a critical place, and contains its fair share of criticism (constructive and destructive) from parents, teachers, critics and competition/audition panels. It has the worst effect of all on the shy personality types who lack the social skills to deal with humiliating put-downs, and such shy people may be in particular danger of systematic mental bullying. A decent assertiveness course is a highly advisable first step for anyone particularly lacking social skills.

Beside this, however, good results in general can be obtained by treating attitude problems in the musical world as 'attributions'. An attribution describes any cause of apparent behaviour that you 'attribute' to somebody or something. Behaviour can be attributed to a set of circumstances ('He's angry because his car was towed away this morning') or to a person's feelings and inner motives ('He's angry because he thinks I can't play the music right'). The problem is where situational reasons are confused with people's motives. We then interpret people's anger as displeasure with us, their tired looks as boredom with us, their failure to make contact as rejection of us. This is known as the 'fundamental attribution error' – that of blaming ourselves for what we assume is our fault, rather than looking for causes outside ourselves, as the following true story illustrates.

A New York singer/actor came on stage just before lunchtime on Friday, the last day of a week of auditioning for a musical. As soon as he reached the front of the stage the producer groaned and said 'Oh no! Not again!' very audibly. The actor fled the stage on the spot, and remained distressed until he happened to meet the producer a few days later.

'How could you humiliate me like that in front of everybody?' he said angrily, recounting what he thought he had witnessed. The producer looked blank for a while, the his face suddenly lit up.

'Oh my God – I know what that was! We'd sent the messenger boy out for some takeaway lunch and told him on no account to bring back the tasteless junk food we'd had all week. I turned round as you came on and saw him coming towards us with yet another pile of junk food takeaways. I must have said 'Oh no! Not again!' pretty loudly – I guess you thought I meant you. Now you mention it, you auditioned very well a few months ago, and we had our eye on you for the part.'

Dealing with attribution errors

Other people's 'vibes', 'attitude problems' or unpredictable behaviour are better dealt with than left in our minds to fester. We have an instinctive feeling that we do not want to deal with 'their stuff', but we may need to really train ourselves to disconnect our own feelings from the moods of others. As little children we will have blamed mummy's bad moods on our 'naughty' behaviour, and we have a lot of unlearning to do to be free of this almost unconscious self-blaming tendency. Steps towards doing this are:

- Remind oneself constantly that there are all sorts of possible reasons for the moods or actions of others. Had the New York actor done that he might have got the part. So don't start with the assumption you are in the wrong.
- Actively try to find out what other people's motivations actually are. Ask them, interpret their actions, look for reasons. Find alternative attributions for your feelings.
- Create 'boundaries' between the moods of others and yourself. See fellow performers as 'inside their skins'. Visualize their whole personality as 'contained' inside their skin, so they stop at the boundary of the skins. They will then seem life-size, and won't 'spill over' towards you. When other people seem negative or critical, this may be a function of their own inability to cope with their problems. People in the grip of inner problems are naturally inflexible, unsociable, defensive or aggressive. By not responding to their bad moods you help them too.
- Be generous to fellow musicians – generosity of spirit is the complete antidote to criticism.

As saxist Cannonball Adderley said: 'fun is what happens when everything is mellow'.

Intrapsychic anxiety

'Performers are egomaniacs with inferiority complexes' is a succinct way of putting it. Musicians, as performers, have two secret fantasies: that they are 'really marvellous' and that they are 'really not that good at all'. How can the musician allow two such irreconcilable fantasies to exist alongside each other? Well, in a variety of clever ways:

- By somehow contriving never to put his talent to the test, by making excuses for instruments, not auditioning for jobs, developing strange physical pains, giving up performing, etc.
- By carrying on playing with some 'excuse' for not doing well, like being drunk, always arriving late, etc.
- By becoming a rebel and maintaining that nobody really understands.
- By convincing himself he is 'a fraud', and suffering constant guilt and anxiety that one day he'll be found out.

This collision of inner fantasies is the reason why the highest stressor in musicians (see Wills and Cooper 1988) is 'feeling you must reach or maintain the standards of musicianship that you set for yourself'. Clearly musicians worry obsessively about their internal standards but carry on performing regardless. The real solution lies in the fact that both these fantasies are some way off reality. Worst fantasies in particular are typically built on things parents or teachers said at some point, such as 'you're too nervous to play in front of audiences' or 'you'll never make it to the big time', which stay in the brain like curses. Such predictors may be totally wrong, and in particular may not allow for the musician's progress over time. A generally more accurate indication of real ability is how other performers value a fellow professional who is getting a reasonable share of work. This reality is a more stable option than the constant roller-coaster of internal fantasies. Who needs fantasies of being 'the best', and who is the 'best' anyway? If the musician is valued by fellow professionals, audiences and pupils enough to stay in the business, then this says a lot.

By 'owning up' to this realistic self-image as others typically see it, the musician can get on with the process of making real gains in his career, rather than forever putting off that wonderful day when 'his talent will be fully revealed to an unsuspecting world'. Fantasy is important to creative artists, such as film-maker Roman Polanski who said one of the secrets of his art was not knowing where reality ended and fantasy started. In the world of Virtual Reality it has been said that 'imagination has replaced money as a unit of currency'. But for the classical musician in particular, reality is a consistent ability to deliver the goods. And the musician is not 'only as good as his last performance' as some would have us believe: he is as good as a lifetime of study and dedication gives him every right to be.

Burnout

I believe that most performers start their love affair with their art form – often at an early age – with somewhere near 100% passion. They then progressively develop from 0% knowledge and disillusionment with the profession to the critical mass of 51% disillusionment. After that the passion for performing goes into negative equity and progressive burnout ensures: performing becomes more disagreeable than agreeable. This is 'spiritual and emotional burnout' (Fig. 1).

Without knowing it, the musician has hit a career plateau where the typical work schedule is fairly similar day in and day out, and this applies as much to international artists as to rank and file performers. Energy of youth burns out revealing any number of underlying tensions, from performing nerves to worry about the future. Ambition gives place to apathy and low performing buzz as careers become more predictable and less varied and challenging.

When burnout is combined with performing anxiety the result is a feeling that 'I can't stand it any more – either I reduce the anxiety or I'm giving my career up just to keep me sane'. Loss of motivation may have caused a fall in professional standards which is bringing the performer down close to the minimum acceptable level.

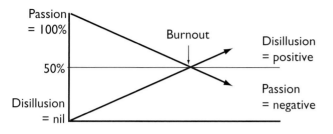

Figure 1

Burnout of primary motivation (passion) over time.

This may have been noticed by others before it really hits the performer. To the performer it may be a sudden awareness that denial is no longer an adequate defence – technical elements are suddenly much harder than they seemed, and there is a realization that one is only just coping. This sudden 'peak' in anxiety may be dramatically worse in performers who have become well known and have heavy schedules in the public eye, sometimes stretching ahead for months and years of advance bookings. Fear may become alarm and the performer fights against a desire to 'call for help', for instance by getting permission from a doctor or other specialist to have a short, long or complete break. Musicians suffering typical symptoms of burnout:

- Don't practise or rehearse enough
- Don't warm up before performances
- Don't listen to other musicians – just try to get their own part right
- Arrive minutes before performance
- Are tempted to or actually read papers/books in rehearsals
- Have stopped doing solo recitals or chamber music
- May feel consuming guilt at falling technical standards, which then turns into stage fright
- May turn up for work drunk or drugged as a way of dealing with nerves
- May use alcohol or cannabis daily and lose track of pressing career needs or reality in general.

Burnout may mirror apathy in other areas (marriage, sex, lapsed hobbies, lapsed sport due to overweight). There may be several common depressive features, such as a sense of 'not looking back to birth but on to death'. Fantasies one wanted to accomplish in one's lifetime may no longer be possible – particularly in career terms. When spirits are low and a career is perceived as hitting a trough, it can share depression's sense of anguish and 'futilitarianism'.

Recovering from burnout

Life on the 'mid-life plateau' can be successfully managed to give variety and enjoyment, but not in the same hectic all-consuming way of the ambitious performer straight out of college, nor in the apathetic and jaded way where actual standards become progressively worse. Increasing passion means reviving interest and commitment, while decreasing disillusionment means managing your life to prioritize pleasure, creativity and variety and decrease all sources of stress. New priorities are:

- Sleep and relaxation: pace work, and make periods of calm around important gigs.
- Regular holidays. Synchronize holidays with your partner where possible. Get help with children so you can get away, e.g. an au-pair.
- Saying no. Eliminate the drudgery of your bottom level of work. Make sure your diary is not overbooked.
- Taking exercise. Be fit for tours which take you into overdrive. Work out or swim.
- Not letting teaching schedules overwhelm you. Organize teaching so it fits you, not the whims and exigencies of your pupils/parents – your own comfort is essential for good teaching.

- Increased communication with other performers and your wider social circle. Keep in touch. Visit friends and vice versa. Have dinner parties.
- Having at least one other passion (hobby, reading, sport etc.) the more interactive the better.
- Increasing the variety of work, e.g. conduct, compose, arrange, broadcast, write articles. Also increase creativity – create your own work rather than relying on others.
- Performing regular solo gigs and playing chamber music with friends.
- Practising for pleasure – take out old pieces as well as your regular exercises.

The team approach to treatment

We have already mentioned some key team members who become involved in all the medical, postural and psychological issues of hand problems. Whether the problem is one of assessment, treatment or rehabilitation – or that of simultaneously treating a physical problem and a general case of performance anxiety – there is an obvious need to compare notes on a shared patient simply to optimize the treatment and impart any extra insights that one or other has obtained. Probably even more important than this is to offer the patient a coherent, believable and co-ordinated treatment plan. It is the patient who is by far the most confused, frustrated and not least out of pocket in being passed around willy nilly from one specialist to the next, and the suffering of the patient should be alleviated as much as possible by clear advice as to who is involved, why they are involved, what can and can't be done, what timescale to expect, and simply how to convert free-floating anxiety and medico-speak overload into a credible recovery plan. If this can include actual practice plans, examinations at regular periods, ongoing psychological support and explanations of what is happening in plain language, so much the better.

I have been very impressed by the work of Dr Richard Norris in the USA in exhaustively analysing the ergonomics of performance and designing recovery programmes that are optimized down to the smallest significant detail. His thoroughness and care is a model for us all; see further Norris (1993).

The concept of the performance psychologist

I have referred to myself throughout as a psychologist rather than a therapist or counsellor for a number of deliberate reasons beyond the fact that I happen to be one by training. In the sense that I have weekly sessions where I sit in a chair and work with musicians I am no different from any other therapist, but the content and approach of such sessions is sometimes radically different from those given by the general therapist, particularly those on the classical psychodynamic model who reveal no personal details and work strictly with transference. For a start, I spend hours talking in great detail about the musician's work, career, instrument, practice plans, performance strategies and inner musical life with an added knowledge that I possess in my other function of being myself a professional musician. I also allow the patient to play their instrument. I listen patiently to CDs and tapes and I try to go to live performances where it helps.

By using the term 'psychologist' I have created an added agenda of trying to introduce musicians to the idea that they have at their disposal just the sort of resource that sportspeople call a 'sport psychologist'. If this serves to enlighten them to the realization that a psychologist is not necessarily someone who sees 'problems' and dwells on 'inefficiency' but a friendly, accessible and expert resource that promotes added 'efficiency', then perhaps more of our musicians will take advantage of all the progress in expert treatment that has been steadily growing over the last decade into a whole new area of professional help that they can be proud of using.

References

Evans A (1994) The Secrets of Musical Confidence. HarperCollins: London.

Freud S, Breuer J (1974) Studies on Hysteria. Penguin Freud Library, vol. 3. Penguin: Harmondsworth.

Norris R (1993) The Musician's Survival Manual: a Guide to Preventing and Treating Injuries in Instrumentalists. Mmb Music: St Louis.

Wills G, Cooper CL (1988) Pressure Sensitive. Sage Publications: London.

17
Medicines and stage fright

Ian James

Excessive anxiety can have a devastating effect on musical performance. For the poor performer it is a nightmare and for the audience who witness it, it is a very uncomfortable experience. Many techniques to cope with the problem have been explored over the centuries, some being more effective than others. Obviously no musician should try and perform something beyond his abilities and everything should be well rehearsed. Despite this many superb and experienced musicians are severely affected by stage fright. Even if the musical performance does not suffer, their health can. Many musicians turn to the medical profession for help. Sadly, the quality of that help can be variable. This review covers the use of medicines to control stage fright, outlining both advantages and disadvantages.

Sedative drugs

There are hundreds of sedative drugs that can be prescribed. Benzodiazepines such as diazepam (Valium) and chlordiazepoxide (Librium) are probably the commonest group to be used. These drugs are widely used to treat generalized anxiety. Their short-term use is often questionable and their long-term use is indefensible. They should not be used for the treatment of stage fright as in this context they are frequently ineffective. In addition, they often have a direct adverse effect on the performance itself by clouding judgement. In the long term (3–4 weeks only) they can provoke addiction and depression. The incidence of usage varies from country to country, being highest in those countries where they are freely available and lowest where they can only be obtained by a doctor's prescription.

Alcohol

Everyone knows that alcohol calms the nerves and bolsters self-esteem. It is therefore popular with musicians and has a specific effect on tremor. It can also cloud judgement and wreck a performance. The dose is, however, an important factor. One or two small drinks taken in a social environment, and not specifically to cure stage fright, may be acceptable. However 'Don't drink and drive' also implies 'Don't drink and play'. Its main danger is that its use can be addictive, and abuse leads to diseases of the liver, heart and nerves. Drinking a large amount of alcohol one evening can lead to a rebound anxiety the next day. The temptation then is to take more alcohol to cope with rebound problems and so the spiral continues.

Beta blockers

Beta blockers, or more correctly beta-adrenergic receptor antagonists, include drugs such as propranolol (Inderal), atenolol, (Tenormin), oxprenolol (Trasicor) and nadolol (Corgard). Their action is to block the effect of adrenaline. Adrenaline is the 'fear hormone' released by the adrenal gland which results in the classic 'fight or flight' response – very useful when confronting a sabre-toothed tiger but of much less use when confronting an audience. The rapid and forceful heartbeat, the trembling of the limbs, the rapid shallow breathing are all caused by adrenaline. Beta blockers have the ability to block these responses. Anxiety is decreased because the physical effects of anxiety are abolished and this is sensed by the brain. It is unlikely that beta-blocking drugs have a direct depressant effect on the brain. In the usual (low) dose there is no intrinsic adverse effect on performance itself. If performance is adversely affected by anxiety that decrement is abolished by the drug. Under these circumstances performance improves. There are numerous scientific studies demonstrating this point.

The improvement in performance applies not only to bow shake or problems with breathing but also to musical aspects such as intonation and phraseing. Beta blockers can precipitate asthma and should never be given to or taken by asthmatics. These drugs should only be taken for specific events and not on a daily basis. Usually they should be taken 1½ hours before performance. The only exception to this is nadolol, which should be taken 4 hours before. Most beta blockers last for 4 hours or so; nadolol lasts for 8–10 hours and has been called the 'Wagner beta blocker'. Atenolol has less effect on tremor than the others and is best avoided in string players. It has been claimed to have less effect on the bronchial tree than other beta blockers but still should never be used in asthmatics. Propranolol is destroyed at a variable rate by the liver and certain factors such as whether one eats prior to a performance can make a great deal of difference to whether the drug works or not. Oxprenolol has a slight adrenaline-like effect of its own, as well as being able to block all the previously mentioned symptoms of fear. The excitement of performance is unimpaired by oxprenolol. Some performers have also reported that it enables them to think more quickly, thereby allowing them to execute those little feats of performance which have been carefully rehearsed but are all too frequently lost in the melée of the event itself. Beta blockers do not make one overvalue one's own performance. In this regard they differ from alcohol, where the reverse is true. If taken in excess beta blockers can slow finger movement. This effect becomes more noticeable at lower temperatures. Some beta blockers can cause a degree of insomnia. Frequently this is not recognized, as the performance itself may also inhibit sleep.

The usage of beta blockers varies from country to country. Where they are freely available some 30% of performers take them on occasion. Where they are available only on a medical prescription the figure is much lower – 10%.

Beta blockers can be used in association with behavioural techniques. This in fact may be the best approach for patients with a chronic stage fright syndrome. The drugs certainly should not be used alone on a daily basis. All players should be warned not to pass beta blockers across the desk to a colleague for he or she may be an asthmatic! Idiosyncratic effects are seen from time to time. It should be emphasized, therefore, that one should first try out the medication on a non-important occasion.

Use in music competitions

It is not for the physician to decide on this question. If the aim of the competition is to assess the best player then there seems no reason why drugs should not be used. If the aim is to find the performer who plays best under the stress of performance then the taking of beta blockers would seem to be unfair.

Depression

It is important to realize that chronic stage fright often leads to depression. Beta blockers do not work under these circumstances. The reasons for this are obscure. The depression must be treated either with drugs such as tricyclic antidepressants (amitriptyline), or 5-hydroxytriptamine-uptake inhibitors (fluoxetine or sertraline), or alternatively by psychotherapy and counselling.

Drugs to avoid

Caffeine contained in coffee, tea and cola can if taken to excess cause tremor and anxiety. All performers should be aware of this. The effect of caffeine gets more marked as one gets older.

Asthmatics who use salbutamol or terbutaline inhalers, especially if they take theophylline-containing medicines as well, become anxious and have tremor. These symptoms are much enhanced by performing. Competent treatment of their asthma, decreasing the troublesome agents and adding others, can often get round the problem.

18
Instrument playing and severe hand deformity

Geoffrey Hooper, Jean Pillet and Helen Scott

Severe deformity of the hand and arm usually results from congenital defect or injury. In either case, the playing of a musical instrument may not be precluded although the youngster with the congenital abnormality will adapt more readily than the adult following injury. For these patients to be successful musically, careful analysis of their deformity must be undertaken and

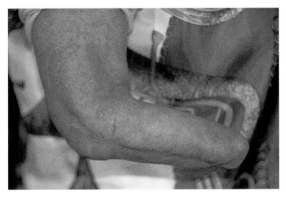

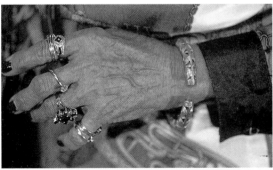

Figure 1

Proximal agenesis (congenital absence of a limb or part of a limb) of the right forearm. This piano teacher won First Prize from the Lyon Conservatory of Music for her interpretation of Ravel's Concerto for the Left Hand; she was fitted with a prosthesis only in 1956, at the age of 40. Since then she has been using her prosthesis every day for social and professional activities but does not wear it either at home or to play the piano.

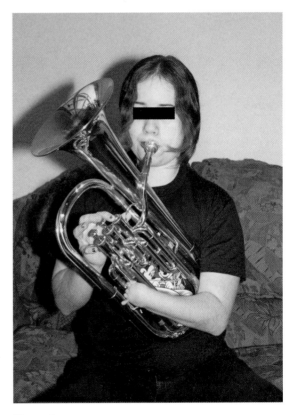

Figure 2

This 20-year-old musician with a left congenital trans-metacarpal deficiency and rudimentary finger nubbins plays the E flat tenor horn using predominantly her normal right hand. She is currently a senior music student at university.

the patient then matched to the instrument, to a suitable prosthesis, to a modified instrument or to combinations of these three factors. Examples of this type of analysis are shown below. For the purposes of analysis, the deformity can be categorized as unilateral or bilateral rather than the more commonly used 'transverse' or 'axial' and the aetiology is irrelevant.

To play with unilateral deformity one may:

• Play single-handedly a usually double-handed instrument (Fig. 1)

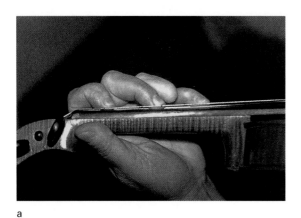

a

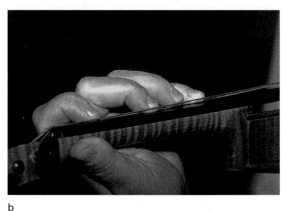

b

Figure 3

No prosthesis, however sophisticated, can replace the human hand. Aesthetic prostheses, in the case of distal finger amputations, make it possible to extend the stump, sometimes providing essential help for musicians. This professional violinist, an accident victim in 1993 at the age of 49, was fitted with a prosthesis in 1994. When playing the violin she always wears her prosthesis but does so very seldom for social activities.

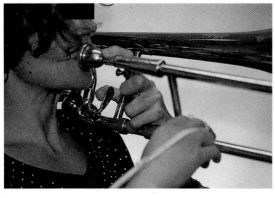

a

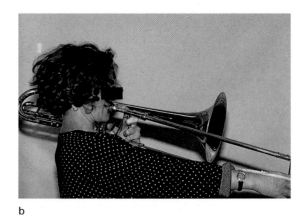

b

Figure 4

Agenetic musicians lead normal lives without any real functional handicap, even if they handle movement differently. They easily adapt to their digital stumps, but in the case of hand or forearm amputations, 'extension prostheses' may be needed to play a musical instrument. Fitted with a prosthesis at the age of 1 in 1958, this professional musician plays the trombone by attaching her prosthetic hand to the slide of her instrument.

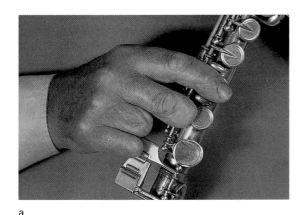

a

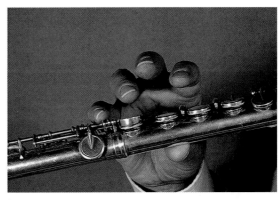

b

Figure 5

In 1983, after an accident at the age of 37, this amateur transverse player was fitted with a prosthesis when he was 57 years old. He only wears the prosthesis when playing this instrument, which was modified in order to stabilize the prosthesis.

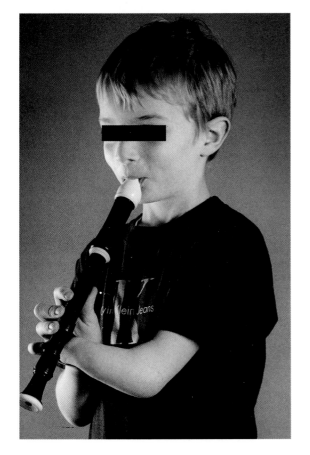

Figure 6

This 6-year-old with agenesis of the right hand plays an Aulos recorder, designed to be played with six digits. In this boy's case the distal left stump functions as the 'sixth' digit operating the lower tone hole on the back of the instrument.

- Play an instrument which effectively requires only one hand (Fig. 2)
- Augment the deformed hand with a prosthesis (Fig. 3)
- Augment with a prosthesis which itself is modified (Fig. 4)
- Augment with a prosthesis and also modify the instrument (Fig. 5)
- Modify the instrument to fit the single-hand deformity (Fig. 6).

To play with bilateral hand deformities one may:

- Reconstruct one hand so the patient may play as a unilateral deformity Fig. 7)

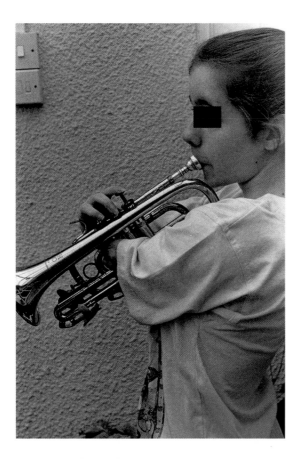

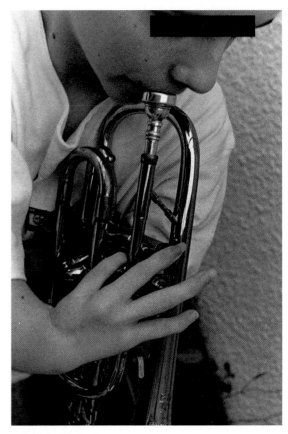

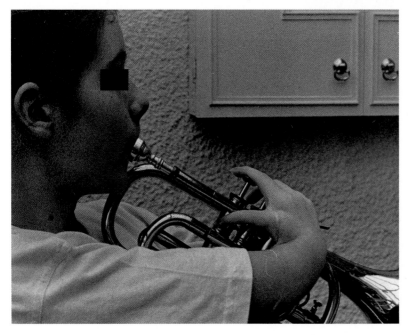

Figure 7

This 15-year-old has almost complete agenesis of the left humerus, a conjoined synostosis of the radius and ulna and a four-digit hand with partial syndactyly on the left, and a radial club hand on the right with partial absence of the radius, a proximal radioulnar synostosis and a four-digit hand reconstructed by pollicization of the right index finger. She plays a normal cornet using her reconstructed right hand to finger and her hypoplastic left upper limb for support. She has achieved school diploma level in this instrument.

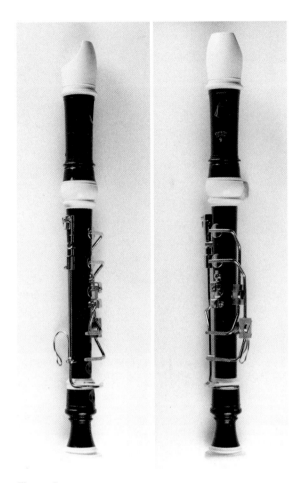

- Use an extensively modified instrument (Fig. 8)

Examples are given where younger players have reached high levels of achievement and older professionals and teachers have been able to maintain their careers even after serious injury.

Figure 8

This highly modified descant recorder is designed to be played with one hand but still have the range of the normal instrument. Additional modifications can be made to accommodate even more severe deformity but the range of the instrument will be reduced.

Appendix I
Bier block

Geoffrey Leader

The traditional technique of intravenous regional anaesthetic block (Bier 1908) has been in use for nearly a century. It is particularly useful for out-patient surgery on the upper extremity (Dunlop 1995) because it fulfils a number of criteria:

- A bloodless field is provided for the surgeon
- The whole arm distal to the tourniquet is analgesic without the need of multiple nerve blocks, or multiple areas of direct infiltration
- There is excellent anaesthesia of bone and joints
- There is a short recovery time and patients can leave the hospital within 1 hour.

In the standard technique (Holmes 1963) a double cuff is placed on the upper arm and intra-venous access is established. An Esmarch bandage is applied to exsanguinate the arm, the upper cuff is inflated above the arterial pressure and 40 ml of ½% lignocaine is injected.

After 10 minutes the lower cuff is inflated and the upper released. The block is tolerated for approximately 35–40 mins. Toxicity is minimal, even when the cuff is released after only 20 minutes. In a series of 500 cases, only 2 patients complained of circumoral tingling and one case suffered from transient faintness with a slight drop in blood pressure.

A modified technique as used in the Hand Clinic, The Devonshire Hospital, London

First modification

Instead of using a double cuff, we place a single cuff on the upper arm, exsanguinate the limb as

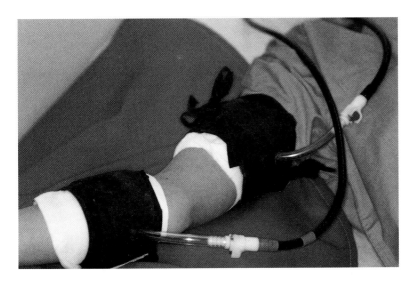

Figure 1

Separate upper and lower arm pneumatic tourniquets used. The distal tourniquet is routinely tolerated without discomfort for 60 minutes.

usual and inject the standard volume of lignocaine. After 10 minutes, the limb distally is exsanguinated by the surgeon using a sterile Esmarch bandage and a lower cuff (Fig. 1), previously placed on the proximal forearm, is inflated. The upper cuff is then deflated.

The advantage of this technique, for example in fracture of the wrist or hand, is that initial exsanguination can be started proximal to the painful fracture site and secondary surgical exsanguination can be performed once that site has become analgesic. Another benefit is that the forearm tourniquet is tolerated for a much longer period than the lower cuff of the double-cuff technique (usually 50–60 minutes). An additional advantage is that in slightly longer procedures we can extend the duration of the block by approximately 15 minutes by alternately inflating and deflating the two cuffs.

We have also noticed that the technique appears to be volume dependent – for large arms therefore we use the same amount of lignocaine diluted to 50–60 ml.

Second modification

After distal exsanguination has been performed we also inject bupivacaine ½% into the skin and subcutaneous tissues at the site of the surgical incision and around the regional nerves where appropriate. This has the advantage of more rapid onset of skin anaesthesia prior to skin incision and of prolonged postoperative analgesia. The modified technique has been used safely and successfully in a combined series of 5000 cases.

Postoperatively the patient is transferred to the recovery room for further monitoring of pulse and blood pressure. Unless sedation has been used, which is unusual, light refreshment may be consumed immediately.

References

Bier A (1908) Ueber einen neuen Weg Localanaesthesie an den Gliedmassen zu erzeugen. *Arch Klin Chir* **86**:1007–16.

Dunlop DJ (1995) The use of Bier block for day surgery. *J Hand Surg* **20B**:679–80.

Holmes CM (1963) Intravenous regional analgesia. A useful method of producing analgesia of the limbs. *Lancet* **1**:245–7.

Appendix II
Thermoplastic splinting materials

Alison T Davis and Gabriele Rogers

There are many different splinting materials available, each with their own characteristic properties and uses. The following list is by no means comprehensive. The materials listed here are the ones the authors use most frequently in their hand clinics.

Orthoplast

- Bright, white matt finish
- Perforated forms available
- Low bulk – light weight
- Semi-rigid, may need reinforcement
- Mouldable in hot water: 72–77°C/hot air
- Modified easily
- Self-bonding when surfaces are hot and dry
- Good malleability: plenty of working time
- Suitable for large splint – does not stretch
- Easy to use – good for less experienced therapist
- Washable; impermeable.

Orfit

- Different types
  - Orfit 'S' – skin (soft and stiff)
  - Orfit 'C'- coated
  - Orfit colours – coloured
- Two levels of mouldability are available
  - soft Orfit: excellent mouldability for producing intricate shapes
  - stiff Orfit: less mouldability but excellent control to cover large areas and general contours
- Four thicknesses: 1.6 mm; 2 mm; 3.2 mm; 4.2 mm
- Four perforations: micro, mini, maxi, non-perforated
- Low bulk – light weight

- Mouldable in hot water: 55–60°C
- Transparent at working temperature
- 100% elastic memory
- Good malleability – suitable for small finger splints
- Need liquid soap in water, cream on patient to prevent sticking
- Difficult to achieve smooth edges
- Washable; impermeable.

Preferred

- Beige
- Perforated forms available
- Low bulk – light weight
- Low rigidity – may need reinforcement
- Mouldable in hot water: 72°C
- Bonds to itself if surface coating is broken or removed
- Has 50% drape and 50% controlled stretch
- Stretch is consistent and will not leave areas of irregular thickness
- Edges bond well when cut with scissors
- Washable; impermeable.

Sansplint polyform

- White
- Perforated forms available
- Low bulk – light weight
- Semi-rigid
- Mouldable in hot water 65°C/hot air
- Self-adheres when hot
- Good malleability with a degree of stretch – needs to be designed and cut undersize to allow for stretch
- Good for creative splinting and small rigid splints
- Washable; impermeable.

X'lite

- White, open mesh
- Semi-rigid and may need reinforcement – usual to work with two layers bonded together
- Low bulk – light weight
- Mouldable in hot water 70°C/hot air
- Modifies easily
- Padding necessary – edges rolled in for smooth finish
- Needs liquid soap in water or cream or gauze on patient to prevent sticking
- Good for open wounds as open mesh allows good ventilation
- Good durability – when layered can be used for heavy uses and weightbearing
- Less easy to wash; impermeable.

Sansplint XR

- White
- Perforated forms available
- Low bulk – light weight
- Semi-rigid; may need reinforcement
- Mouldable in hot water 65°C/hot air
- Self-adheres when hot
- Very good malleability – large degree of stretch and conforms around awkward curves/contours
- Suitable for intricate hand splints
- Marks easily with thumbprints
- Not suitable for inexperienced therapist due to large degree of drape/stretch
- Washable; impermeable.

Index